Virtual Clinical Excursions—General Hospital

for

Potter and Perry:
Basic Nursing,
7th Edition

prepared by

Patricia A. Potter, RN, MSN, PhD, FAAN
Research Scientist
Siteman Cancer Center at Barnes-Jewish Hospital and
Washington University School of Medicine
St. Louis, Missouri

Anne Griffin Perry, RN, EdD, FAAN
Professor and Associate Dean
School of Nursing
Southern Illinois University Edwardsville
Edwardsville, Illinois

Kim D. Cooper, RN, MSN
Ivy Tech Community College
Terre Haute, Indiana

software developed by

Wolfsong Informatics, LLC
Tucson, Arizona

ELSEVIER
MOSBY

3251 Riverport Lane
Maryland Heights, Missouri 63043

VIRTUAL CLINICAL EXCURSIONS—GENERAL HOSPITAL FOR
POTTER AND PERRY: BASIC NURSING,
SEVENTH EDITION

ISBN: 978-0-323-07390-5

Copyright © 2011, 2007 by Mosby, Inc., an affiliate of Elsevier Inc.

Notice

ISBN: 978-0-323-07390-5

Executive Editor: *Tom Wilhelm*
Managing Editor: *Jeff Downing*
Associate Developmental Editor: *Krissy Prysmiki*
Project Manager: *Joy Moore*

**Working together to grow
libraries in developing countries**

www.elsevier.com | www.bookaid.org | www.sabre.org

ELSEVIER   BOOK AID International   Sabre Foundation

Printed in the United States of America

Last digit is the print number: 9 8 7 6 5 4 3 2

Virtual Clinical Excursions—General Hospital

for

Potter and Perry:
Basic Nursing,
7th Edition

Workbook
prepared by

Patricia A. Potter, RN, MSN, PhD, FAAN
Research Scientist
Siteman Cancer Center at Barnes-Jewish Hospital and
Washington University School of Medicine
St. Louis, Missouri

Anne Griffin Perry, RN, EdD, FAAN
Professor and Associate Dean
School of Nursing
Southern Illinois University Edwardsville
Edwardsville, Illinois

Kim D. Cooper, RN, MSN
Ivy Tech Community College
Terre Haute, Indiana

Textbook

Patricia A. Potter, RN, MSN, PhD, FAAN
Research Scientist
Siteman Cancer Center at Barnes-Jewish Hospital and
Washington University School of Medicine
St. Louis, Missouri

Anne Griffin Perry, RN, EdD, FAAN
Professor and Associate Dean
School of Nursing
Southern Illinois University Edwardsville
Edwardsville, Illinois

Contents

Getting Started

Part I—Application of Nursing Concepts

Part II—Clinical Care of Patients

Part III—Psychosocial Care in Practice

Table of Contents
Potter and Perry
Basic Nursing, 7th Edition

Getting Started

GETTING SET UP

■ MINIMUM SYSTEM REQUIREMENTS

WINDOWS®

Windows Vista®, XP, 2000 (Recommend Windows XP/2000)
Pentium® III processor (or equivalent) @ 600 MHz (Recommend 800 MHz or better)
256 MB of RAM (Recommend 1 GB or more for Windows Vista)
800 x 600 screen size (Recommend 1024 x 768)
Thousands of colors
12x CD-ROM drive
Soundblaster 16 soundcard compatability
Stereo speakers or headphones

Note: Windows Vista and XP require administrator privileges for installation.

MACINTOSH®

MAC OS X (up to 10.6.1)
Apple Power PC G3 @ 500 MHz or better
128 MB of RAM (Recommend 256 MB or more)
800 x 600 screen size (Recommend 1024 x 768)
Thousands of colors
12x CD-ROM drive
Stereo speakers or headphones

■ INSTALLATION INSTRUCTIONS

WINDOWS

1. Insert the *Virtual Clinical Excursions—General Hospital* CD-ROM.
2. The setup screen should appear automatically if the current product is not already installed. Windows Vista users may be asked to authorize additional security prompts.
3. Follow the onscreen instructions during the setup process.

   If the setup screen does *not* appear automatically (and *Virtual Clinical Excursions— General Hospital* has not been installed already):
   a. Click the **My Computer** icon on your desktop or on your Start menu.
   b. Double-click on your CD-ROM drive.
   c. If installation does not start at this point:
      (1) Click the **Start** icon on the taskbar and select the **Run** option.
      (2) Type d:\setup.exe (where "d:\" is your CD-ROM drive) and press **OK**.
      (3) Follow the onscreen instructions for installation.

MACINTOSH

1. Insert the *Virtual Clinical Excursions—General Hospital* CD in the CD-ROM drive. The disk icon will appear on your desktop.

2. Double-click on the disk icon.

3. Double-click on the VCEGENERAL_MAC run file.

Note: Virtual Clinical Excursions—General Hospital for Macintosh does not have an installation setup and can only be run directly from the CD.

■ HOW TO USE VIRTUAL CLINICAL EXCURSIONS—GENERAL HOSPITAL

WINDOWS

1. Double-click on the *Virtual Clinical Excursions—General Hospital* icon located on your desktop.
2. Or navigate to the program via the Windows Start menu.

Note: If your computer uses Windows Vista, right-click on the desktop shortcut and choose **Properties**. In the Compatibility Mode, check the box for "Run as Administrator." Below is a screen capture to show what this looks like.

MACINTOSH

1. Insert the *Virtual Clinical Excursions—General Hospital* CD in the CD-ROM drive. The disk icon will appear on your desktop.

2. Double-click on the disk icon.

3. Double-click on the VCEGENERAL_MAC run file.

■ SCREEN SETTINGS

For best results, your computer monitor resolution should be set at a minimum of 800 x 600. The number of colors displayed should be set to "thousands or higher" (High Color or 16 bit) or "millions of colors" (True Color or 24 bit).

Windows

1. From the **Start** menu, select **Control Panel** (on some systems, you will first go to **Settings**, then to **Control Panel**).
2. Double-click on the **Display** icon.
3. Click on the **Settings** tab.
4. Under **Screen resolution** use the slider bar to select **800 by 600 pixels**.
5. Access the **Colors** drop-down menu by clicking on the down arrow.
6. Select **High Color (16 bit)** or **True Color (24 bit)**.
7. Click on **OK**.
8. You may be asked to verify the setting changes. Click **Yes**.
9. You may be asked to restart your computer to accept the changes. Click **Yes**.

Macintosh

1. Select the **Monitors** control panel.
2. Select **800 x 600** (or similar) from the **Resolution** area.
3. Select **Thousands** or **Millions** from the **Color Depth** area.

■ WEB BROWSERS

Supported web browsers include Microsoft Internet Explorer (IE) version 7.0 or higher or Mozilla 3.0 or higher.

If you use America Online® (AOL) for web access, you will need AOL version 4.0 or higher and one of the browsers listed above. Do not use earlier versions of AOL with earlier versions of IE, because you will have difficulty accessing many features.

For best results with AOL:
- Connect to the Internet using AOL version 4.0 or higher.
- Open a private chat within AOL (this allows the AOL client to remain open, without asking whether you wish to disconnect while minimized).
- Minimize AOL.
- Launch a recommended browser.

■ TECHNICAL SUPPORT

Technical support for this product is available 24 hours a day, seven days a week, excluding holidays. Before calling, be sure that your computer meets the minimum system requirements to run this software. Inside the United States and Canada, call 1-800-222-9570. Outside North America, call 314-447-8094. You may also fax your questions to 314-447-8078 or contact Technical Support through e-mail: technical.support@elsevier.com.

Trademarks: Windows, Macintosh, Pentium, and America Online are registered trademarks.

Copyright © 2011, 2007 by Mosby, Inc., an affiliate of Elsevier Inc.

All rights reserved. No part of this product may be reproduced or transmitted in any form or by any means, electronic or mechanical, including input or storage in any information system, without written permission from the publisher.

ACCESSING *Virtual Clinical Excursions—General Hospital* FROM EVOLVE

The product you have purchased is part of the Evolve family of online courses and learning resources. Please read the following information thoroughly to get started.

To access your instructor's course on Evolve:

Your instructor will provide you with the username and password needed to access this specific course on the Evolve Learning System. Once you have received this information, please follow these instructions:

1. Go to the Evolve student page (http://evolve.elsevier.com/student).

2. Enter your username and password in the **Login to My Evolve** area and click the **Login** button.

3. You will be taken to your personalized **My Evolve** page, where the course will be listed in the **My Courses** module.

TECHNICAL REQUIREMENTS

To use an Evolve course, you will need access to a computer that is connected to the Internet and equipped with web browser software that supports frames. For optimal performance, it is recommended that you have speakers and use a high-speed Internet connection. However, slower dial-up modems (56 K minimum) are acceptable.

Whichever browser you use, the browser preferences must be set to enable cookies and the cache must be set to reload every time.

Enable Cookies

Browser	Steps
Internet Explorer (IE) 7.0 or higher	1. Select **Tools → Internet Options**. 2. Select **Privacy** tab. 3. Use the slider (slide down) to **Accept All Cookies**. 4. Click **OK**. -OR- 3. Click the **Advanced** button. 4. Click the check box next to **Override Automatic Cookie Handling**. 5. Click the **Accept** radio buttons under **First-party Cookies** and **Third-party Cookies**. 6. Click **OK**.
Mozilla Firefox 3.0 or higher	1. Select **Tools → Options**. 2. Select the **Privacy** icon. 3. Click to expand Cookies. 4. Select **Allow sites to set cookies**. 5. Click **OK**.

Set Cache to Always Reload a Page

Browser	Steps
Internet Explorer (IE) 7.0 or higher	1. Select **Tools → Internet Options**. 2. Select **General** tab. 3. Go to the **Temporary Internet Files** and click the **Settings** button. 4. Select the radio button for **Every visit to the page** and click **OK** when complete.
Mozilla Firefox 3.0 or higher	1. Select **Tools → Options**. 2. Select the **Privacy** icon. 3. Click to expand Cache. 4. Set the value to "**0**" in the **Use up to: __ MB of disk space for the cache** field. 5. Click **OK**.

Plug-Ins

Adobe Acrobat Reader—With the free Acrobat Reader software, you can view and print Adobe PDF files. Many Evolve products offer student and instructor manuals, checklists, and more in this format!

Download at: http://www.adobe.com

Apple QuickTime—Install this to hear word pronunciations, heart and lung sounds, and many other helpful audio clips within Evolve Online Courses!

Download at: http://www.apple.com

Adobe Flash Player—This player will enhance your viewing of many Evolve web pages, as well as educational short-form to long-form animation within the Evolve Learning System!

Download at: http://www.adobe.com

Adobe Shockwave Player—Shockwave is best for viewing the many interactive learning activities within Evolve Online Courses!

Download at: http://www.adobe.com

Microsoft Word Viewer—With this viewer, Microsoft Word users can share documents with those who don't have Word, and users without Word can open and view Word documents. Many Evolve products have testbank, student and instructor manuals, and other documents available for downloading and viewing on your own computer!

Download at: http://www.microsoft.com

Microsoft PowerPoint Viewer—With this viewer, you can access PowerPoint 97, 2000, and 2002 presentations even if you don't have PowerPoint. Many Evolve products have slides available for downloading and viewing on your own computer!

Download at: http://www.microsoft.com

SUPPORT INFORMATION

Live phone support is available to customers in the United States and Canada at **800-222-9570** 24 hours a day, seven days a week. Support is also available through email at technical.support@elsevier.com.

Online 24/7 support can be accessed on the Evolve website (http://evolve.elsevier.com). Resources include:

- Guided tours
- Tutorials
- Frequently asked questions (FAQs)
- Online copies of course user guides
- And much more!

A QUICK TOUR

Welcome to *Virtual Clinical Excursions—General Hospital*, a virtual hospital setting in which you can work with multiple complex patient simulations and also learn to access and evaluate the information resources that are essential for high-quality patient care. The virtual hospital, Pacific View Regional Hospital, has realistic architecture and access to patient rooms, a Nurses' Station, and a Medication Room.

■ BEFORE YOU START

Make sure you have your textbook nearby when you use the *Virtual Clinical Excursions— General Hospital* CD. You will want to consult topic areas in your textbook frequently while working with the CD and using this workbook.

■ HOW TO SIGN IN

- Enter your name on the Student Nurse identification badge.
- Next, specify the floor on which you will work by clicking the down arrow next to **Select Floor**. For this quick tour, choose **Medical-Surgical**.
- Now click the down arrow next to **Select Period of Care**. This drop-down menu gives you four periods of care from which to choose. In Periods of Care 1 through 3, you can actively engage in patient assessment, entry of data in the electronic patient record (EPR), and medication administration. Period of Care 4 presents the day in review. Highlight and click the appropriate period of care. (For this quick tour, choose **Period of Care 1: 0730-0815**.)
- Click **Go**. This takes you to the Patient List screen (see example on page 11). Note that the virtual time is provided in the box at the lower left corner of the screen (0730, since we chose Period of Care 1).

Note: If you choose to work during Period of Care 4: 1900-2000, the Patient List screen is skipped since you are not able to visit patients or administer medications during the shift. Instead, you are taken directly to the Nurses' Station, where the records of all the patients on the floor are available for your review.

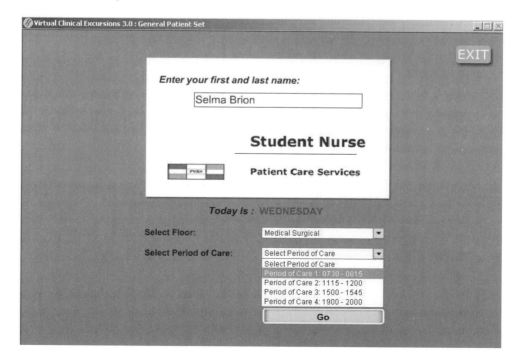

■ PATIENT LIST

MEDICAL-SURGICAL UNIT

Harry George (Room 401)

Osteomyelitis—A 54-year-old Caucasian male admitted from a homeless shelter with an infected leg. He has complications of type 2 diabetes mellitus, alcohol abuse, nicotine addiction, poor pain control, and complex psychosocial issues.

Jacquline Catanazaro (Room 402)

Asthma—A 45-year-old Caucasian female admitted with an acute asthma exacerbation and suspected pneumonia. She has complications of chronic schizophrenia, noncompliance with medication therapy, obesity, and herniated disc.

Piya Jordan (Room 403)

Bowel obstruction—A 68-year-old Asian female admitted with a colon mass and suspected adenocarcinoma. She undergoes a right hemicolectomy. This patient's complications include atrial fibrillation, hypokalemia, and symptoms of meperidine toxicity.

Clarence Hughes (Room 404)

Degenerative joint disease—A 73-year-old African-American male admitted for a left total knee replacement. His preparations for discharge are complicated by the development of a pulmonary embolus and the need for ongoing intravenous therapy.

Pablo Rodriguez (Room 405)

Metastatic lung carcinoma—A 71-year-old Hispanic male admitted with symptoms of dehydration and malnutrition. He has chronic pain secondary to multiple subcutaneous skin nodules and psychosocial concerns related to family issues with his approaching death.

Patricia Newman (Room 406)

Pneumonia—A 61-year-old Caucasian female admitted with worsening pulmonary function and an acute respiratory infection. Her chronic emphysema is complicated by heavy smoking, hypertension, and malnutrition. She needs access to community resources such as a smoking cessation program and meal assistance.

SKILLED NURSING UNIT

William Jefferson (Room 501)

Alzheimer's disease—A 75-year-old African-American male admitted for stabilization of type 2 diabetes and hypertension following a recent acute care admission for a urinary tract infection and sepsis. His complications include episodes of acute delirium and a history of osteoarthritis.

Kathryn Doyle (Room 503)

Rehabilitation post left hip replacement—A 79-year-old Caucasian female admitted following a complicated recovery from an ORIF. She is experiencing symptoms of malnutrition and depression due to unstable family dynamics, placing her at risk for elder abuse.

Goro Oishi (Room 505)

Hospice care—A 66-year-old Asian male admitted following an acute care admission for an intracerebral hemorrhage and resulting coma. Family-staff interactions provide opportunities to explore death and dying issues related to conflict about advanced life support and cultural and religious differences.

OBSTETRICS UNIT

Dorothy Grant (Room 201)

30-week intrauterine pregnancy—A 25-year-old multipara admitted with abdominal trauma following a domestic violence incident. Her complications include preterm labor and extensive social issues such as acquiring safe housing for her family upon discharge.

■ HOW TO SELECT A PATIENT

- You can choose one or more patients to work with from the Patient List by checking the box to the left of the patient name(s). For this quick tour, select Piya Jordan and Pablo Rodriguez. (In order to receive a scorecard for a patient, the patient must be selected before proceeding to the Nurses' Station.)
- Click on **Get Report** to the right of the medical records number (MRN) to view a summary of the patient's care during the 12-hour period before your arrival on the unit.
- After reviewing the report, click on **Go to Nurses' Station** in the right lower corner to begin your care. (*Note:* If you have been assigned to care for multiple patients, you can click on **Return to Patient List** to select and review the report for each additional patient before going to the Nurses' Station.)

Note: Even though the Patient List is initially skipped when you sign in to work for Period of Care 4, you can still access this screen if you wish to review the shift report for any of the patients. To do so, simply click on **Patient List** near the top left corner of the Nurses' Station (or click on the clipboard to the left of the Kardex). Then click on **Get Report** for the patient(s) whose care you are reviewing. This may be done during any period of care.

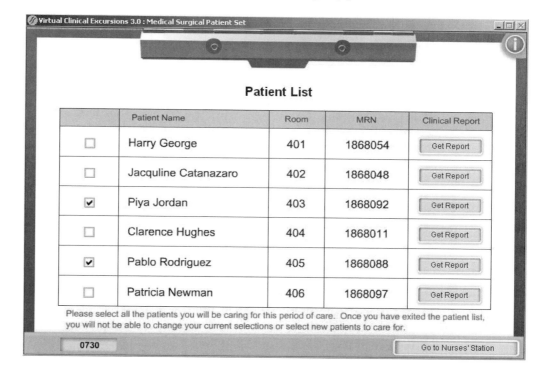

■ HOW TO FIND A PATIENT'S RECORDS

NURSES' STATION

Within the Nurses' Station, you will see:

1. A clipboard that contains the patient list for that floor.
2. A chart rack with patient charts labeled by room number, a notebook labeled Kardex, and a notebook labeled MAR (Medication Administration Record).
3. A desktop computer with access to the Electronic Patient Record (EPR).
4. A tool bar across the top of the screen that can also be used to access the Patient List, EPR, Chart, MAR, and Kardex. This tool bar is also accessible from each patient's room.
5. A Drug Guide containing information about the medications you are able to administer to your patients.
6. A tool bar across the bottom of the screen that can be used to access the Floor Map, patient rooms, Medication Room, and Drug Guide.

As you run your cursor over an item, it will be highlighted. To select, simply double-click on the item. As you use these resources, you will always be able to return to the Nurses' Station by clicking on the **Return to Nurses' Station** bar located in the right lower corner of your screen.

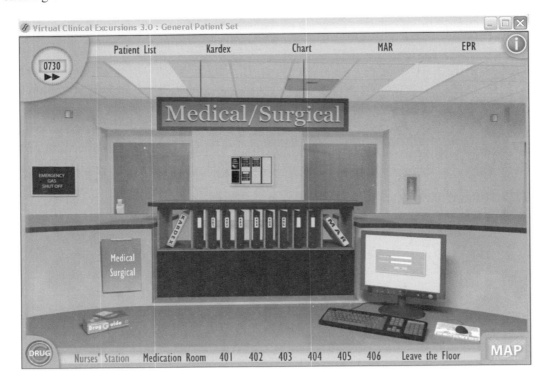

MEDICATION ADMINISTRATION RECORD (MAR)

The MAR icon located on the tool bar at the top of your screen accesses current 24-hour medications for each patient. Click on the icon and the MAR will open. (*Note:* You can also access the MAR by clicking on the MAR notebook on the far right side of the book rack in the center of the screen.) Within the MAR, tabs on the right side of the screen allow you to select patients by room number. Be careful to make sure you select the correct tab number for *your* patient rather than simply reading the first record that appears after the MAR opens. Each MAR sheet lists the following:

- Medications
- Route and dosage of each medication
- Times of administration of each medication

Note: The MAR changes each day. Expired MARs are stored in the patients' charts.

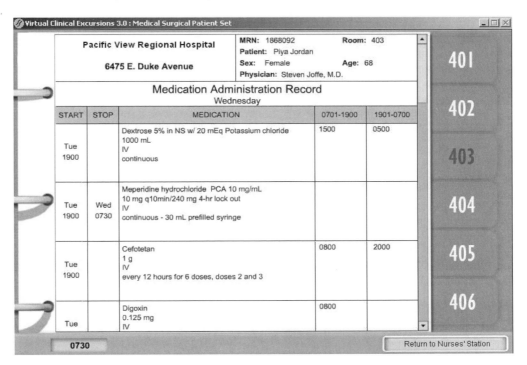

CHARTS

To access patient charts, either click on the **Chart** icon at the top of your screen or anywhere within the chart rack in the center of the Nurses' Station screen. When the close-up view appears, the individual charts are labeled by room number. To open a chart, click on the room number of the patient whose chart you wish to review. The patient's name and allergies will appear on the left side of the screen, along with a list of tabs on the right side of the screen, allowing you to view the following data:

- Allergies
- Physician's Orders
- Physician's Notes
- Nurse's Notes
- Laboratory Reports
- Diagnostic Reports
- Surgical Reports
- Consultations

- Patient Education
- History and Physical
- Nursing Admission
- Expired MARs
- Consents
- Mental Health
- Admissions
- Emergency Department

Information appears in real time. The entries are in reverse chronologic order, so use the down arrow at the right side of each chart page to scroll down to view previous entries. Flip from tab to tab to view multiple data fields or click on **Return to Nurses' Station** in the lower right corner of the screen to exit the chart.

ELECTRONIC PATIENT RECORD (EPR)

The EPR can be accessed from the computer in the Nurses' Station or from the EPR icon located in the tool bar at the top of your screen. To access a patient's EPR:
- Click on either the computer screen or the **EPR** icon.
- Your username and password are automatically filled in.
- Click on **Login** to enter the EPR.
- *Note:* Like the MAR, the EPR is arranged numerically. Thus when you enter, you are initially shown the records of the patient in the lowest room number on the floor. To view the correct data for *your* patient, remember to select the correct room number, using the drop-down menu for the Patient field at the top left corner of the screen.

The EPR used in Pacific View Regional Hospital represents a composite of commercial versions being used in hospitals. You can access the EPR:
- to review existing data for a patient (by room number).
- to enter data you collect while working with a patient.

The EPR is updated daily, so no matter what day or part of a shift you are working, there will be a current EPR with the patient's data from the past days of the current hospital stay. This type of simulated EPR allows you to examine how data for different attributes have changed over time, as well as to examine data for all of a patient's attributes at a particular time. The EPR is fully functional (as it is in a real-life hospital). You can enter such data as blood pressure, breath sounds, and certain treatments. The EPR will not, however, allow you to enter data for a previous time period. Use the arrows at the bottom of the screen to move forward and backward in time.

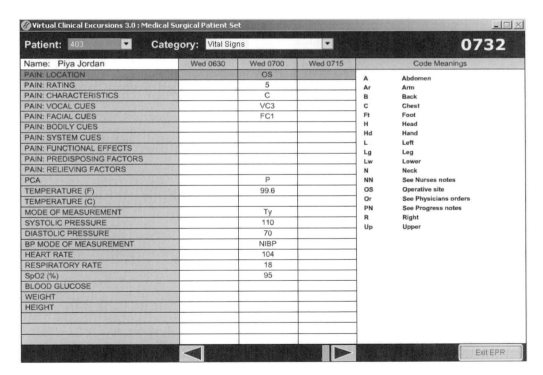

Name: Piya Jordan	Wed 0630	Wed 0700	Wed 0715	Code Meanings	
PAIN: LOCATION		OS		A	Abdomen
PAIN: RATING		5		Ar	Arm
PAIN: CHARACTERISTICS		C		B	Back
PAIN: VOCAL CUES		VC3		C	Chest
PAIN: FACIAL CUES		FC1		Ft	Foot
PAIN: BODILY CUES				H	Head
PAIN: SYSTEM CUES				Hd	Hand
PAIN: FUNCTIONAL EFFECTS				L	Left
PAIN: PREDISPOSING FACTORS				Lg	Leg
PAIN: RELIEVING FACTORS				Lw	Lower
PCA		P		N	Neck
TEMPERATURE (F)		99.6		NN	See Nurses notes
TEMPERATURE (C)				OS	Operative site
MODE OF MEASUREMENT		Ty		Or	See Physicians orders
SYSTOLIC PRESSURE		110		PN	See Progress notes
DIASTOLIC PRESSURE		70		R	Right
BP MODE OF MEASUREMENT		NIBP		Up	Upper
HEART RATE		104			
RESPIRATORY RATE		18			
SpO2 (%)		95			
BLOOD GLUCOSE					
WEIGHT					
HEIGHT					

At the top of the EPR screen, you can choose patients by their room numbers. In addition, you have access to 17 different categories of patient data. To change patients or data categories, click the down arrow to the right of the room number or category.

The categories of patient data in the EPR are as follows:

- Vital Signs
- Respiratory
- Cardiovascular
- Neurologic
- Gastrointestinal
- Excretory
- Musculoskeletal
- Integumentary
- Reproductive
- Psychosocial
- Wounds and Drains
- Activity
- Hygiene and Comfort
- Safety
- Nutrition
- IV
- Intake and Output

Remember, each hospital selects its own codes. The codes used in the EPR at Pacific View Regional Hospital may be different from ones you have seen in your clinical rotations. Take some time to acquaint yourself with the codes. Within the Vital Signs category, click on any item in the left column (e.g., Pain: Characteristics). In the far-right column, you will see a list of code meanings for the possible findings and/or descriptors for that assessment area.

You will use the codes to record the data you collect as you work with patients. Click on the box in the last time column to the right of any item and wait for the code meanings applicable to that entry to appear. Select the appropriate code to describe your assessment findings and type it in the box. (*Note:* If no cursor appears within the box, click on the box again until the blue shading disappears and the blinking cursor appears.) Once the data are typed in this box, they are entered into the patient's record for this period of care only.

To leave the EPR, click on **Exit EPR** in the bottom right corner of the screen.

■ VISITING A PATIENT

From the Nurses' Station, click on the room number of the patient you wish to visit (in the tool bar at the bottom of your screen). Once you are inside the room, you will see a still photo of your patient in the top left corner. To verify that this is the correct patient, click on the **Check Armband** icon to the right of the photo. The patient's identification data will appear. If you click on **Check Allergies** (the next icon to the right), a list of the patient's allergies (if any) will replace the photo.

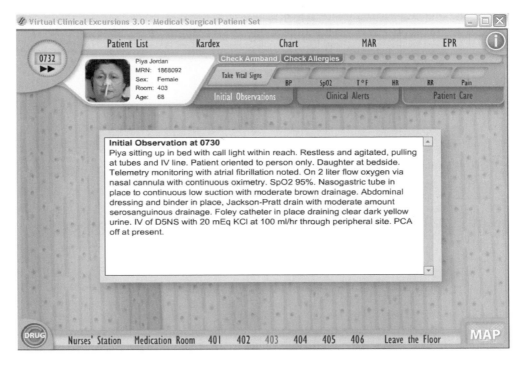

Also located in the patient's room are multiple icons you can use to assess the patient or the patient's medications. A virtual clock is provided in the upper left corner of the room to monitor your progress in real time. (*Note:* The fast-forward icon within the virtual clock will advance the time by 2-minute intervals when clicked.)

- The tool bar across the top of the screen allows you to check the **Patient List**, access the **EPR** to check or enter data, and view the patient's **Chart**, **MAR**, or **Kardex**.

- The **Take Vital Signs** icon allows you to measure the patient's up-to-the-minute blood pressure, oxygen saturation, temperature, heart rate, respiratory rate, and pain level.

- Each time you enter a patient's room, you are given an Initial Observation report to review (in the text box under the patient's photo). These notes are provided to give you a "look" at the patient as if you had just stepped into the room. You can also click on the **Initial Observations** icon to return to this box from other views within the patient's room. To the right of this icon is **Clinical Alerts**, a resource that allows you to make decisions about priority medication interventions based on emerging data collected in real time. Check this screen throughout your period of care to avoid missing critical information related to recently ordered or STAT medications.

- Clicking on **Patient Care** opens up three specific learning environments within the patient room: **Physical Assessment**, **Nurse-Client Interactions**, and **Medication Administration**.

- To perform a **Physical Assessment**, choose a body area (such as **Head & Neck**) from the column of yellow buttons. This activates a list of system subcategories for that body area (e.g., see **Sensory**, **Neurologic**, etc. in the green boxes). After you select the system you wish to evaluate, a brief description of the assessment findings will appear in a box to the right. A still photo provides a "snapshot" of how an assessment of this area might be done or what the finding might look like. For every body area, you can also click on **Equipment** on the right side of the screen.

- To the right of the Physical Assessment icon is **Nurse-Client Interactions**. Clicking on this icon will reveal the times and titles of any videos available for viewing. (*Note:* If the video you wish to see is not listed, this means you have not yet reached the correct virtual time to view that video. Check the virtual clock; you may return to access the video once its designated time has occurred—as long as you do so within the same period of care. Or you can click on the fast-forward icon within the virtual clock to advance the time by 2-minute intervals. You will then need to click again on **Patient Care** and **Nurse-Client Interactions** to refresh the screen.) To view a listed video, click on the white arrow to the right of the video title. Use the control buttons below the video to start, stop, pause, rewind, or fast-forward the action or to mute the sound.

- **Medication Administration** is the pathway that allows you to review and administer medications to a patient after you have prepared them in the Medication Room. This process is addressed further in the *How to Prepare Medications* section (pages 19-20) and in *Medications* (pages 26-30). For additional hands-on practice, see *Reducing Medication Errors* (pages 37-41).

■ HOW TO QUIT, CHANGE PATIENTS, CHANGE FLOORS, OR CHANGE PERIODS OF CARE

How to Quit: From most screens, you may click the **Leave the Floor** icon on the bottom tool bar to the right of the patient room numbers. (*Note:* From some screens, you will first need to click an **Exit** button or **Return to Nurses' Station** before clicking **Leave the Floor**.) When the Floor Menu appears, click **Exit** to leave the program.

How to Change Patients, Floors, or Periods of Care: To change patients, simply click on the new patient's room number. (You cannot receive a scorecard for a new patient, however, unless you have already selected that patient on the Patient List screen.) To change to a new period of care, to change floors, or to restart the virtual clock, click on **Leave the Floor** and then on **Restart the Program**.

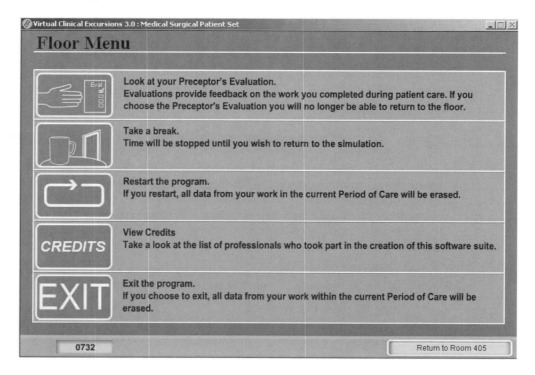

■ HOW TO PREPARE MEDICATIONS

From the Nurses' Station or the patient's room, you can access the Medication Room by clicking on the icon in the tool bar at the bottom of your screen to the left of the patient room numbers.

In the Medication Room you have access to the following (from left to right):

- A preparation area is located on the counter under the cabinets. To begin the medication preparation process, click on the tray on the counter or click on the **Preparation** icon at the top of the screen. The next screen leads you through a specific sequence (called the Preparation Wizard) to prepare medications one at a time for administration to a patient. However, no medication has been selected at this time. We will do this while working with a patient in *A Detailed Tour*. To exit this screen, click on **View Medication Room**.

- To the right of the cabinets (and above the refrigerator), IV storage bins are provided. Click on the bins themselves or on the **IV Storage** icon at the top of the screen. The bins are labeled **Microinfusion**, **Small Volume**, and **Large Volume**. Click on an individual bin to see a list of its contents. If you needed to prepare an IV medication at this time, you could click on the medication and its label would appear to the right under the patient's name. (*Note:* You can **Open** and **Close** any medication label by clicking the appropriate icon.) Next, you would click **Put Medication on Tray**. If you ever change your mind or decide that you have put the incorrect medication on the tray, you can reverse your actions by highlighting the medication on the tray and then clicking **Put Medication in Bin**. Click **Close Bin** in the right bottom corner to exit. **View Medication Room** brings you back to a full view of the entire room.

- A refrigerator is located under the IV storage bins to hold any medications that must be stored below room temperature. Click on the refrigerator door or on the **Refrigerator** icon at the top of the screen. Then click on the close-up view of the door to access the medications. When you are finished, click **Close Door** and then **View Medication Room**.

- To prepare controlled substances, click the **Automated System** icon at the top of the screen or click the computer monitor located to the right of the IV storage bins. A login screen will appear; your name and password are automatically filled in. Click **Login**. Select the patient for whom you wish to access medications; then select the correct medication drawer to open (they are stored alphabetically). Click **Open Drawer**, highlight the proper medication, and choose **Put Medication on Tray**. When you are finished, click **Close Drawer** and then **View Medication Room**.

- Next to the Automated System is a set of drawers identified by patient room number. To access these, click on the drawers or on the **Unit Dosage** icon at the top of the screen. This provides a close-up view of the drawers. To open a drawer, click on the room number of the patient you are working with. Next, click on the medication you would like to prepare for the patient, and a label will appear, listing the medication strength, units, and dosage per unit. To exit, click **Close Drawer**; then click **View Medication Room**.

At any time, you can learn about a medication you wish to prepare for a patient by clicking on the **Drug** icon in the bottom left corner of the medication room screen or by clicking the **Drug Guide** book on the counter to the right of the unit dosage drawers. The **Drug Guide** provides information about the medications commonly included in nursing drug handbooks. Nutritional supplements and maintenance intravenous fluid preparations are not included. Highlight a medication in the alphabetical list; relevant information about the drug will appear in the screen below. To exit, click **Return to Medication Room**.

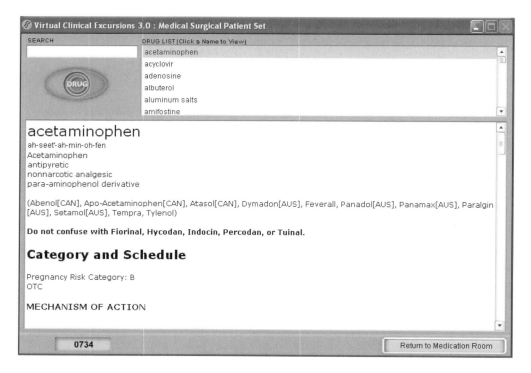

To access the MAR to review the medications ordered for a patient, click on the **MAR** icon located in the tool bar at the top of your screen and then click on the correct tab for your patient's room number. You may also click the **Review MAR** icon in the tool bar at the bottom of your screen from inside each medication storage area.

After you have chosen and prepared medications, go to the patient's room to administer them by clicking on the room number in the bottom tool bar. Inside the patient's room, click **Patient Care** and then **Medication Administration** and follow the proper administration sequence.

■ PRECEPTOR'S EVALUATIONS

When you have finished a session, click on **Leave the Floor** to go to the Floor Menu. At this point, you can click on the top icon (**Look at Your Preceptor's Evaluation**) to receive a score-card that provides feedback on the work you completed during patient care.

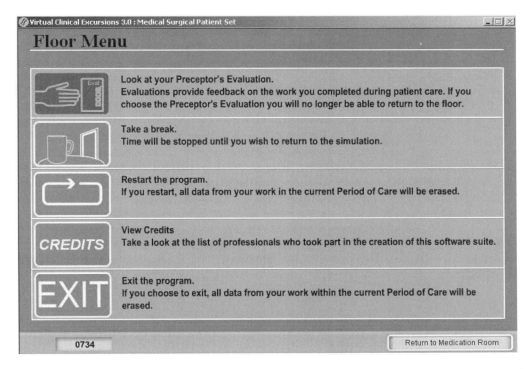

Evaluations are available for each patient you selected when you signed in for the current period of care. Click on the **Medication Scorecard** icon to see an example.

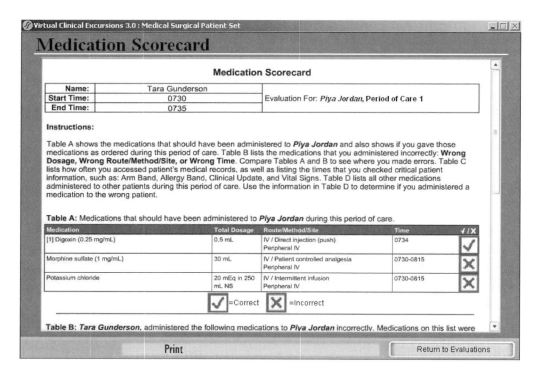

The scorecard compares the medications you administered to a patient during a period of care with what should have been administered. Table A lists the correct medications. Table B lists any medications that were administered incorrectly.

Remember, not every medication listed on the MAR should necessarily be given. For example, a patient might have an allergy to a drug that was ordered, or a medication might have been improperly transcribed to the MAR. Predetermined medication "errors" embedded within the program challenge you to exercise critical thinking skills and professional judgment when deciding to administer a medication, just as you would in a real hospital. Use all your available resources, such as the patient's chart and the MAR, to make your decision.

Table C lists the resources that were available to assist you in medication administration. It also documents whether and when you accessed these resources. For example, did you check the patient armband or perform a check of vital signs? If so, when?

You can click **Print** to get a copy of this report if needed. When you have finished reviewing the scorecard, click **Return to Evaluations** and then **Return to Menu**.

■ FLOOR MAP

To get a general sense of your location within the hospital, you can click on the **Map** icon found in the lower right corner of most of the screens in the *Virtual Clinical Excursions—General Hospital* program. (*Note:* If you are following this quick tour step by step, you will need to **Restart the Program** from the Floor Menu, sign in again, and go to the Nurses' Station to access the map.) When you click the **Map** icon, a floor map appears, showing the layout of the floor you are currently on, as well as a directory of the patients and services on that floor. As you move your cursor over the directory list, the location of each room is highlighted on the map (and vice versa). The floor map can be accessed from the Nurses' Station, Medication Room, and each patient's room.

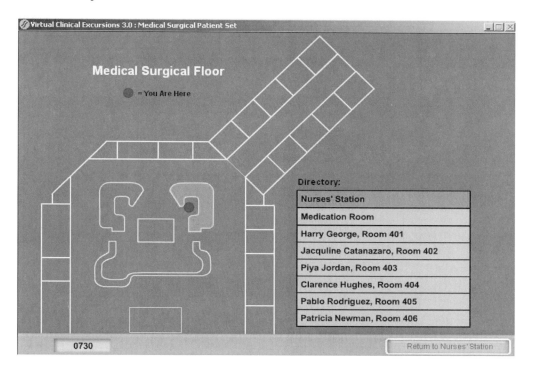

A DETAILED TOUR

If you wish to more thoroughly understand the capabilities of *Virtual Clinical Excursions— General Hospital*, take a detailed tour by completing the following section. During this tour, we will work with a specific patient to introduce you to all the different components and learning opportunities available within the software.

■ WORKING WITH A PATIENT

Sign in and select the Medical-Surgical Floor for Period of Care 1 (0730-0815). From the Patient List, select Piya Jordan and Pablo Rodriguez; however, do not go to the Nurses' Station yet.

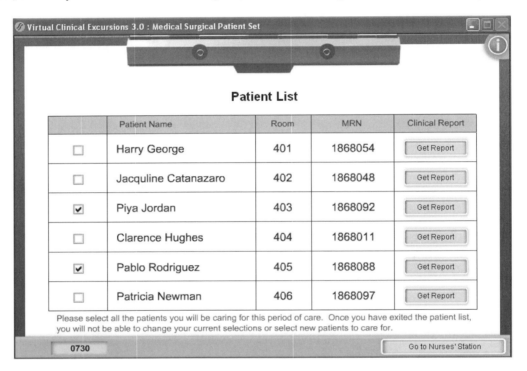

■ REPORT

In hospitals, when one shift ends and another begins, the outgoing nurse who attended a patient will give a verbal and sometimes a written summary of that patient's condition to the incoming nurse who will assume care for the patient. This summary is called a report and is an important source of data to provide an overview of a patient. Your first task is to get the clinical report on Piya Jordan. To do this, click **Get Report** in the far right column in this patient's row. From a brief review of this summary, identify the problems and areas of concern that you will need to address for this patient.

When you have finished noting any areas of concern, click on **Go to Nurses' Station**.

■ CHARTS

You can access Piya Jordan's chart from the Nurses' Station or from the patient's room (403). From the Nurses' Station, click on the chart rack or on the **Chart** icon in the tool bar at the top of your screen. Next, click on the chart labeled **403** to open the medical record for Piya Jordan. Click on the **Emergency Department** tab to view a record of why this patient was admitted.

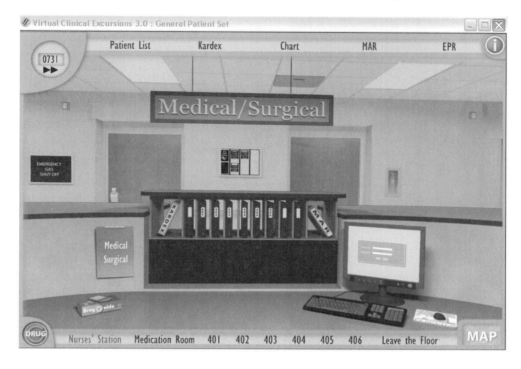

How many days has Piya Jordan been in the hospital?

What tests were done upon her arrival in the Emergency Department and why?

What was her reason for admission?

You should also click on **Surgical Reports** to learn what procedures were performed and when. Finally, review the **Nursing Admission** and **History and Physical** to learn about the health history of this patient. When you are done reviewing the chart, click **Return to Nurses' Station**.

■ MEDICATIONS

Open the Medication Administration Record (MAR) by clicking on the **MAR** icon in the tool bar at the top of your screen. *Remember:* The MAR automatically opens to the first occupied room number on the floor—which is not necessarily your patient's room number! Since you need to access Piya Jordan's MAR, click on tab **403** (her room number). Always make sure you are giving the *Right Drug to the Right Patient!*

Examine the list of medications ordered for Piya Jordan. In the table below, list the medications that need to be given during this period of care (0730-0815). For each medication, note the dosage, route, and time to be given.

Time	Medication	Dosage	Route

Click on **Return to Nurses' Station**. Next, click on **403** on the bottom tool bar and then verify that you are indeed in Piya Jordan's room. Select **Clinical Alerts** (the icon to the right of Initial Observations) to check for any emerging data that might affect your medication administration priorities. Next, go to the patient's chart (click on the **Chart** icon; then click on **403**). When the chart opens, select the **Physician's Orders** tab.

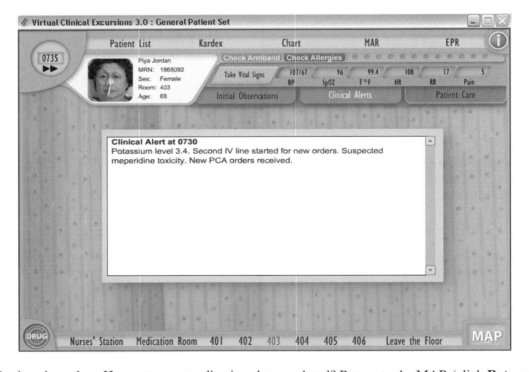

Review the orders. Have any new medications been ordered? Return to the MAR (click **Return to Room 403**; then click **MAR**). Verify that the new medications have been correctly transcribed to the MAR. Mistakes are sometimes made in the transcription process in the hospital setting, and it is sound practice to double-check any new order.

Are there any patient assessments you will need to perform before administering these medications? If so, return to Room 403 and click on **Patient Care** and then **Physical Assessment** to complete those assessments before proceeding.

Now click on the **Medication Room** icon in the tool bar at the bottom of your screen to locate and prepare the medications for Piya Jordan.

In the Medication Room, you must access the medications for Piya Jordan from the specific dispensing system in which each medication is stored. Locate each medication that needs to be given in this time period and click on **Put Medication on Tray** as appropriate. (*Hint:* Look in **Unit Dosage** drawer first.) When you are finished, click on **Close Drawer** and then on **View Medication Room**. Now click on the medication tray on the counter on the left side of the medication room screen to begin preparing the medications you have selected. (*Remember:* You can also click **Preparation** in the tool bar at the top of the screen.)

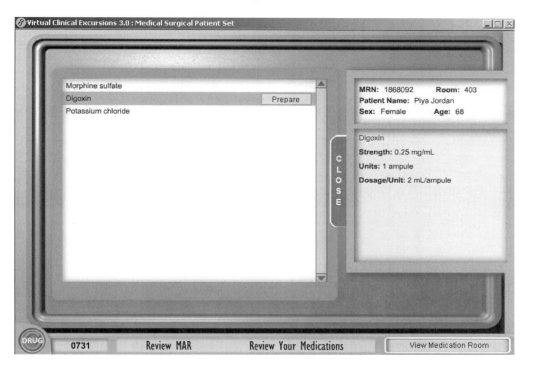

In the preparation area, you should see a list of the medications you put on the tray in the previous steps. Click on the first medication and then click **Prepare**. Follow the onscreen instructions of the Preparation Wizard, providing any data requested. As an example, let's follow the preparation process for digoxin, one of the medications due to be administered to Piya Jordan during this period of care. To begin, click to select **Digoxin**; then click **Prepare**. Now work through the Preparation Wizard sequence as detailed below:

Amount of medication in the ampule: 2 mL.
Enter the amount of medication you will draw up into a syringe: **0.5** mL.
Click **Next**.
Select the patient you wish to set aside the medication for: **Room 403, Piya Jordan**.
Click **Finish**.
Click **Return to Medication Room**.

Follow this same basic process for the other medications due to be administered to Piya Jordan during this period of care. (*Hint:* Look in **IV Storage** and **Automated System**.)

PREPARATION WIZARD EXCEPTIONS

- Some medications in *Virtual Clinical Excursions—General Hospital* are prepared by the pharmacy (e.g., IV antibiotics) and taken to the patient room as a whole. This is common practice in most hospitals.
- Blood products are not administered by students through the *Virtual Clinical Excursions—General Hospital* simulations since blood administration follows specific protocols not covered in this program.
- The *Virtual Clinical Excursions—General Hospital* simulations do not allow for mixing more than one type of medication, such as regular and Lente insulins, in the same syringe. In the clinical setting, when multiple types of insulin are ordered for a patient, the regular insulin is drawn up first, followed by the longer-acting insulin. Insulin is always administered in a special unit-marked syringe.

Now return to Room 403 (click on **403** on the bottom tool bar) to administer Piya Jordan's medications.

At any time during the medication administration process, you can perform a further review of systems, take vital signs, check information contained within the chart, or verify patient identity and allergies. Inside Piya Jordan's room, click **Take Vital Signs**. (*Note:* These findings change over time to reflect the temporal changes you would find in a patient similar to Piya Jordan.)

When you have gathered all the data you need, click on **Patient Care** and then select **Medication Administration**. Any medications you prepared in the previous steps should be listed on the left side of your screen. Let's continue the administration process with the digoxin ordered for Piya Jordan. Click to highlight **Digoxin** in the list of medications. Next, click on the down arrow to the right of **Select** and choose **Administer** from the drop-down menu. This will activate the Administration Wizard. Complete the Wizard sequence as follows:

- Route: **IV**
- Method: **Direct Injection**
- Site: **Peripheral IV**
- Click **Administer to Patient** arrow.
- Would you like to document this administration in the MAR? **Yes**
- Click **Finish** arrow.

Your selections are recorded by a tracking system and evaluated on a Medication Scorecard stored under Preceptor's Evaluations. This scorecard can be viewed, printed, and given to your instructor. To access the Preceptor's Evaluations, click on **Leave the Floor**. When the Floor Menu appears, select **Look at Your Preceptor's Evaluation**. Then click on **Medication Scorecard** inside the box with Piya Jordan's name (see example on the following page).

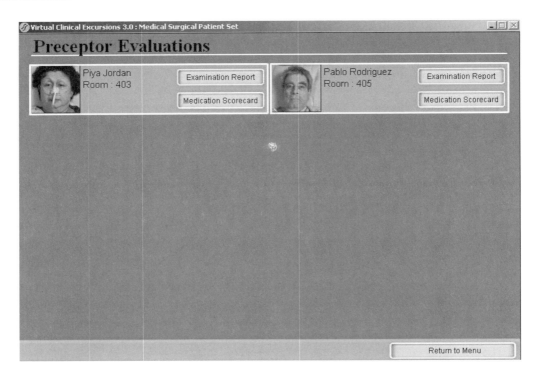

■ MEDICATION SCORECARD

- First, review Table A. Was digoxin given correctly? Did you give the other medications as ordered?
- Table B shows you which (if any) medications you gave incorrectly.
- Table C addresses the resources used for Piya Jordan. Did you access the patient's chart, MAR, EPR, or Kardex as needed to make safe medication administration decisions?
- Did you check the patient's armband to verify her identity? Did you check whether your patient had any known allergies to medications? Were vital signs taken?

When you have finished reviewing the scorecard, click **Return to Evaluations** and then **Return to Menu**.

■ VITAL SIGNS

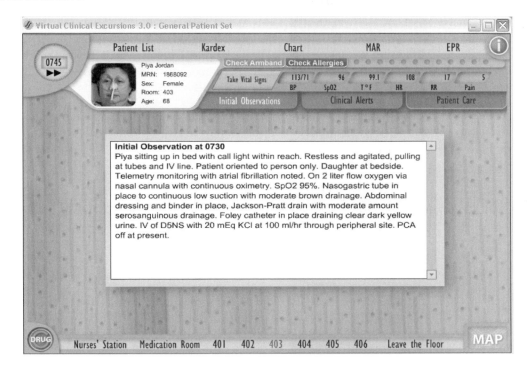

Vital signs, often considered the traditional "signs of life," include body temperature, heart rate, respiratory rate, blood pressure, oxygen saturation of the blood, and pain level.

Inside Piya Jordan's room, click **Take Vital Signs**. (*Note:* If you are following this detailed tour step by step, you will need to **Restart the Program** from the Floor Menu, sign in again, and navigate to Room 403.) Collect vital signs for this patient and record them below. Note the time at which you collected each of these data. (*Remember:* You can take vital signs at any time. The data change over time to reflect the temporal changes you would find in a patient similar to Piya Jordan.)

Vital Signs	Findings/Time
Blood pressure	
O$_2$ saturation	
Heart rate	
Respiratory rate	
Temperature	
Pain rating	

After you are done, click on the **EPR** icon located in the tool bar at the top of the screen. Your username and password are automatically provided. Click on **Login** to enter the EPR. To access Piya Jordan's records, click on the down arrow next to Patient and choose her room number, **403**. Select **Vital Signs** as the category. Next, in the empty time column on the far right, record the vital signs data you just collected in Piya Jordan's room. (*Note:* If you need help with this process, see page 16.) Now compare these findings with the data you collected earlier for this patient's vital signs. Use these earlier findings to establish a baseline for each of the vital signs.

    a.   Are any of the data you collected significantly different from the baseline for a particular vital sign?

        Circle One: Yes   No

    b.   If "Yes," which data are different?

■ PHYSICAL ASSESSMENT

After you have finished examining the EPR for vital signs, click **Exit EPR** to return to Room 403. Click **Patient Care** and then **Physical Assessment**. Think about the information you received in the report at the beginning of this shift, as well as what you may have learned about this patient from the chart. Based on this, what area(s) of examination should you pay most attention to at this time? Is there any equipment you should be monitoring? Conduct a physical assessment of the body areas and systems that you consider priorities for Piya Jordan. For example, select **Head & Neck**; then click on and assess **Sensory** and **Lymphatic**. Complete any other assessment(s) you think are necessary at this time. In the following table, record the data you collected during this examination.

Area of Examination	Findings
Head & Neck Sensory	
Head & Neck Lymphatic	

After you have finished collecting these data, return to the EPR. Compare the data that were already in the record with those you just collected.

    a.   Are any of the data you collected significantly different from the baselines for this patient?

        Circle One: Yes   No

    b.   If "Yes," which data are different?

■ NURSE-CLIENT INTERACTIONS

Click on **Patient Care** from inside Piya Jordan's room (403). Now click on **Nurse-Client Interactions** to access a short video titled **Pain—Adverse Drug Event**, which is available for viewing at or after 0735 (based on the virtual clock in the upper left corner of your screen; see *Note* below.). To begin the video, click on the white arrow next to its title. You will observe a nurse communicating with Piya Jordan and her daughter. There are many variations of nursing practice, some exemplifying "best" practice and some not. Note whether the nurse in this interaction displays professional behavior and compassionate care. Are her words congruent with what is going on with the patient? Does this interaction "feel right" to you? If not, how would you handle this situation differently? Explain.

Note: If the video you wish to view is not listed, this means you have not yet reached the correct virtual time to view that video. Check the virtual clock; you may return to access the video once its designated time has occurred—as long as you do so within the same period of care. Or you can click on the fast-forward icon within the virtual clock to advance the time by 2-minute intervals. You will then need to click again on **Patient Care** and **Nurse-Client Interactions** to refresh the screen.

At least one Nurse-Client Interactions video is available during each period of care. Viewing these videos can help you learn more about what is occurring with a patient at a certain time and also prompt you to discern between nurse communications that are ideal and those that need improvement. Compassionate care and the ability to communicate clearly are essential components of delivering quality nursing care, and it is during your clinical time that you will begin to refine these skills.

■ COLLECTING AND EVALUATING DATA

Each of the activities you perform in the Patient Care environment generates a significant amount of assessment data. Remember that after you collect data, you can record your findings in the EPR. You can also review the EPR, patient's chart, videos, and MAR at any time. You will get plenty of practice collecting and then evaluating data in context of the patient's course.

Now, here's an important question for you:

> Did the previous sequence of exercises provide the most efficient way to assess Piya Jordan?

For example, you went to the patient's room to get vital signs, then back to the EPR to enter data and compare your findings with extant data. Next, you went back to the patient's room to do a physical examination, then again back to the EPR to enter and review data. If this back-and-forth process of data collection and recording seemed inefficient, remember the following:

- Plan all of your nursing activities to maximize efficiency, while at the same time optimizing the quality of patient care. (Think about what data you might need before performing certain tasks. For example, do you need to check a heart rate before administering a cardiac medication or check an IV site before starting an infusion?)

- You collect a tremendous amount of data when you work with a patient. Very few people can accurately remember all these data for more than a few minutes. Develop efficient assessment skills, and record data as soon as possible after collecting them.

- Assessment data are only the starting point for the nursing process.

Make a clear distinction between these first exercises and how you actually provide nursing care. These initial exercises were designed to involve you actively in the use of different software components. This workbook focuses on sensible practices for implementing the nursing process in ways that ensure the highest-quality care of patients.

Most important, remember that a human being changes through time, and that these changes include both the physical and psychosocial facets of a person as a living organism. Think about this for a moment. Some patients may change physically in a very short time (a patient with emerging myocardial infarction) or more slowly (a patient with a chronic illness). Patients' overall physical and psychosocial conditions may improve or deteriorate. They may have effective coping skills and familial support, or they may feel alone and full of despair. In fact, each individual is a complex mix of physical and psychosocial elements, and at least some of these elements usually change through time.

Thus it is crucial that you *DO NOT* think of the nursing process as a simple one-time, five-step procedure consisting of assessment, nursing diagnosis, planning, implementation, and evaluation. Rather, the nursing process should be utilized as a creative and systematic approach to delivering nursing care. Furthermore, because all living organisms are constantly changing, we must apply the nursing process over and over. Each time we follow the nursing process for an individual patient, we refine our understanding of that patient's physical and psychosocial conditions based on collection and analysis of many different types of data. *Virtual Clinical Excursions—General Hospital* will help you develop both the creativity and the systematic approach needed to become a nurse who is equipped to deliver the highest-quality care to all patients.

REDUCING MEDICATION ERRORS

Earlier in this detailed tour, you learned the basic steps of medication preparation and administration. The following simulations will allow you to practice those skills further—with an increased emphasis on reducing medication errors by using the Medication Scorecard to evaluate your work.

Sign in to work on the Medical-Surgical Floor at Pacific View Regional Hospital for Period of Care 1. (*Note:* If you are already working with another patient or during another period of care, click on **Leave the Floor** and then **Restart the Program**; then sign in.)

From the Patient List, select Clarence Hughes. Then click on **Go to Nurses' Station**. Complete the following steps to prepare and administer medications to Clarence Hughes.

- Click on **Medication Room**.
- Click on **MAR** and then on tab **404** to determine prn medications that have been ordered for Clarence Hughes. (*Note:* You may click on **Review MAR** at any time to verify the correct medication order. Always remember to check the patient name on the MAR to make sure you have the correct patient's record—you must click on the correct room number tab within the MAR.) Click on **Return to Medication Room** after reviewing the correct MAR.
- Click on **Unit Dosage** (or on the Unit Dosage cabinet); from the close-up view, click on drawer **404**.
- Select the medications you would like to administer. After each selection, click **Put Medication on Tray**. When you are finished selecting medications, click **Close Drawer** and then **View Medication Room**.
- Click **Automated System** (or on the Automated System unit itself). Click **Login**.
- On the next screen, specify the correct patient and drawer location.
- Select the medication you would like to administer and click **Put Medication on Tray**. Repeat this process if you wish to administer other medications from the Automated System.
- When you are finished, click **Close Drawer** and **View Medication Room**.
- From the Medication Room, click **Preparation** (or on the preparation tray).
- From the list of medications on your tray, highlight the correct medication to administer and click **Prepare**.
- This activates the Preparation Wizard. Supply any requested information; then click **Next**.
- Now select the correct patient to receive this medication and click **Finish**.
- Repeat the previous three steps until all medications that you want to administer are prepared.
- You can click on **Review Your Medications** and then on **Return to Medication Room** when ready. Once you are back in the Medication Room, go directly to Clarence Hughes' room by clicking on **404** at the bottom of the screen.
- Inside the patient's room, administer the medication, utilizing the six rights of medication administration. After you have collected the appropriate assessment data and are ready for administration, click **Patient Care** and then **Medication Administration**. Verify that the correct patient and medication(s) appear in the left-hand window. Highlight the first medication you wish to administer; then click the down arrow next to Select. From the drop-down menu, select **Administer** and complete the Administration Wizard by providing any information requested. When the Wizard stops asking for information, click **Administer to Patient**. Specify **Yes** when asked whether this administration should be recorded in the MAR. Finally, click **Finish**.

■ **SELF-EVALUATION**

Now let's see how you did during your medication administration!

- Click on **Leave the Floor** at the bottom of your screen. From the Floor Menu, select **Look at Your Preceptor's Evaluation**. Then click **Medication Scorecard**.

The following exercises will help you identify medication errors, investigate possible reasons for these errors, and reduce or prevent medication errors in the future.

1. Start by examining Table A. These are the medications you should have given to Clarence Hughes during this period of care. If each of the medications in Table A has a ✓ by it, then you made no errors. Congratulations!

If any medication has an X by it, then you made one or more medication errors.

Compare Tables A and B to determine which of the following types of errors you made: Wrong Dose, Wrong Route/Method/Site, or Wrong Time. Follow these steps:
   a. Find medications in Table A that were given incorrectly.
   b. Now see if those same medications are in Table B, which shows what you actually administered to Clarence Hughes.
   c. Comparing Tables A and B, match the Strength, Dose, Route/Method/Site, and Time for each medication you administered incorrectly.
   d. Then, using the form below, list the medications given incorrectly and mark the errors you made for each medication.

Medication	Strength	Dosage	Route	Method	Site	Time
	❑	❑	❑	❑	❑	❑
	❑	❑	❑	❑	❑	❑
	❑	❑	❑	❑	❑	❑
	❑	❑	❑	❑	❑	❑

2. To help you reduce future medication errors, consider the following list of possible reasons for errors.

- Did not check drug against MAR for correct patient, correct date, correct time, correct drug, and correct dose.
- Did not check drug dose against MAR three times.
- Did not open the unit dose package in the patient's room.
- Did not correctly identify the patient using two identifiers.
- Did not administer the drug on time.
- Did not verify patient allergies.
- Did not check the patient's current condition or vital sign parameters.
- Did not consider why the patient would be receiving this drug.
- Did not question why the drug was in the patient's drawer.
- Did not check the physician's order and/or check with the pharmacist when there was a question about the drug or dose.
- Did not verify that no adverse effects had occurred from a previous dose.

Based on the list of possibilities you just reviewed, determine how you made each error and record the reason in the form below:

Medication	Reason for Error

3. Look again at Table B. Are there medications listed that are not in Table A? If so, you gave a medication to Clarence Hughes that he should not have received. Complete the following exercises to help you understand how such an error might have been made.

   a. Perhaps you gave a medication that was on Clarence Hughes' MAR for this period of care, without recognizing that a change had occurred in the patient's condition, which should have caused you to reconsider. Review patient records as necessary and complete the following form:

Medication	Possible Reasons Not to Give This Medication

   b. Another possibility is that you gave Clarence Hughes a medication that should have been given at a different time. Check his MAR and complete the form below to determine whether you made a Wrong Time error:

Medication	Given to Clarence Hughes at What Time	Should Have Been Given at What Time

c. Maybe you gave another patient's medication to Clarence Hughes. In this case, you made a Wrong Patient error. Check the MARs of other patients and use the form below to determine whether you made this type of error:

Medication	Given to Clarence Hughes	Should Have Been Given to

4. The Medication Scorecard provides some other interesting sources of information. For example, if there is a medication selected for Clarence Hughes but it was not given to him, there will be an X by that medication in Table A, but it will not appear in Table B. In that case, you might have given this medication to some other patient, which is another type of Wrong Patient error. To investigate further, look at Table D, which lists the medications you gave to other patients. See whether you can find any medications ordered for Clarence Hughes that were given to another patient by mistake. However, before you make any decisions, be sure to cross-check the MAR for other patients because the same medication may have been ordered for multiple patients. Use the following form to record your findings:

Medication	Should Have Been Given to Clarence Hughes	Given by Mistake to

5. Now take some time to review the medication exercises you just completed. Use the form below to create an overall analysis of what you have learned. Once again, record each of the medication errors you made, including the type of each error. Then, for each error you made, indicate specifically what you would do differently to prevent this type of error from occurring again.

Medication	Type of Error	Error Prevention Tactic

Submit this form to your instructor if required as a graded assignment, or simply use these exercises to improve your understanding of medication errors and how to reduce them.

Name: _____   Date: _____

The following icons are used throughout this workbook to help you quickly identify particular activities and assignments:

 Indicates a reading assignment—tells you which textbook chapter(s) you should read before starting each lesson

 Indicates a writing activity

 Marks the beginning of an interactive CD-ROM activity—signals you to open or return to your *Virtual Clinical Excursions—General Hospital* CD-ROM

 Indicates additional CD-ROM instructions

 Indicates questions and activities that require you to consult your textbook

 Indicates the approximate time required to complete an exercise

LESSON **1**

Critical Thinking and Nursing Judgment

Reading Assignment: Critical Thinking (Chapter 7)
Nursing Process (Chapter 8)
Pain Management (Chapter 31)

Patient: Harry George, Medical-Surgical Floor, Room 401

Objectives:

- Identify how to apply critical thinking to the assessment of a patient.
- Discuss ways to use reflection when preparing for patient care.
- Identify examples of critical thinking attitudes applied in the assessment of patients in the case studies.
- Describe how intellectual standards apply in patient assessment.
- Identify examples of professional standards to use in patient care.
- Apply a critical thinking model to the assessment of patients in the case studies.

Overview:

Each patient experience poses new opportunities and problems involving patient care. In each clinical situation, you have the responsibility to think critically and make sound clinical decisions. During any patient encounter, you must use the skills of critical thinking: applying the nursing process, recalling past experiences that can help in the care of your current patient, reflecting on the knowledge that applies to a patient's health situation, applying intellectual standards and critical thinking attitudes, and exercising professional standards of practice.

The challenge of clinical decision making is rewarding and fulfilling. Each patient presents a unique clinical picture that requires you to observe and examine the patient closely, search for patterns of patient problems, consider scientific principles relating to patient problems, recognize the problems and develop a plan of care, and then act on the plan and evaluate results. Ultimately, the use of critical thinking in patient care enables you to find the solutions that best support and help your patient toward an improved level of health.

Exercise 1

 CD-ROM Activity

 45 minutes

In this exercise you will visit Harry George, a 54-year-old Caucasian male who was admitted to the hospital with symptoms of infection and swelling of the foot. Harry George has a history of abusing alcohol. He has been diagnosed with cellulitis and osteomyelitis of the foot. You may have worked with Harry George previously if you already completed Lesson 16, 17, or 18.

- Sign in to work at Pacific View Regional Hospital on the Medical-Surgical Floor for Period of Care 1. (*Note:* If you are already in the virtual hospital from a previous exercise, click on **Leave the Floor** and then **Restart the Program** to get to the sign-in window.)
- From the Patient List, select Harry George (Room 401).
- Click on **Get Report**.
- Click on **Go to Nurses' Station**.
- Click on **Chart** and then on **401**.
- Click on **Nursing Admission** and review the information provided.

1. Fill in the following form by completing each category as you review the Nursing Admission history for Harry George.

Reason for Admission/Chief Complaint
Nutrition/Metabolic
Skin
Activity/Rest
Self-Perception
Pain

• Review the nurse's admission description of the patient's left leg wound.
 • Next, click on **Consultations** and review the note from the wound care team.

2. Intellectual standards of critical thinking are commonly applied when assessing a patient. Compare the description of Harry George's left foot in the Nursing Admission with the description in the Wound Care Team Consult.

 a. Which note was more complete? Explain.

 b. The wound care team reported the wound at 3 cm, whereas the nurse's note reported 2 cm. How would you validate the assessment finding?

 c. In what way was the Wound Care Team Consult note more precise?

 3. What objective professional standard was used in the assessment of Harry George's pain? (*Study Tip:* Review pages 879-885 in your textbook.)

4. After collecting assessment data and validating for accuracy, you begin to interpret the clinical information by organizing it into meaningful:
 a. inferences.
 b. problems.
 c. clusters.
 d. nursing diagnoses.

 • Click on **Return to Nurses' Station**.
 • Click on **EPR** and **Login**.
 • Specify **401** from the Patient drop-down menu and then select **Vital Signs** from the Category drop-down menu.
 • Review the data from Monday at 1835 to Wednesday 0700.
 • Now select **Nutrition** from the Category drop-down menu and review the data for the same time frame.

5. Certain cues will usually alert you to patterns that suggest a nursing diagnosis. Based on the data you have reviewed in the Nursing Admission and EPR, match each defining characteristic below with its corresponding data from Harry George's admission history.

Defining Characteristic	Admission Data
_____ Verbal report	a. Change in sleep cycle
_____ Sore, inflamed buccal cavity	b. Groans
_____ Lack of interest in food	c. Eats one meal a day
_____ Expressive behavior	d. "My foot is killing me"
_____ Sleep disturbance	e. Gums dark pink, swollen
_____ Reported food intake less than RDA	f. "Haven't felt like eating for last week"

6. As a nurse puts together cues, patterns emerge in the form of nursing diagnoses. Sometimes cues for more than one nursing diagnosis overlap. In the case of Harry George, his sleep disturbance might indicate the effects of the diagnosis Pain, or this could be a defining characteristic for the diagnosis Disturbed Sleep Pattern. As a critical thinker, what would you do to clarify and to be sure data were interpreted correctly?

7. As the nurse, you review the Activity/Rest portion of the Nursing Admission history. The sleep pattern is documented as being "irregular, never more than 2 hours." Your decision to question the patient further about the sleep habits he follows—time he normally goes to bed, activities before going to sleep, and number of awakenings during night—is an example of what critical thinking attitude?
   a. Humility
   b. Thinking independently
   c. Risk taking
   d. Perseverance

 • Click on **Exit EPR**.
   • Click on **Chart** and then **401**.
   • Click on **History and Physical** and review.
   • Find and review the physician's plan.

8. Critical thinking involves the application of knowledge in order to fully analyze and understand a patient's problems. Given the physician's medical plan, list four areas of knowledge that would help you in supporting the plan of care.

• Click on **Return to Nurses' Station**.
   • Select **401** at the bottom of the screen to visit the patient's room.
   • Click on **Patient Care**.
   • Select **Lower Extremities** and review the assessment findings.

In each of the following questions, fill in the blank with the critical thinking concept that best describe the situation.

9. After you review the condition of Harry George's wound, the conclusion as to whether the

   wound is healing is an example of _____ _____.

10. When you see a change in a wound from reddened margins to clear and less inflamed, you

    make a(n) _____ from this evidence in order to conclude that the wound is healing.

11. After you apply saline to Harry George's wound for 2 days, your evaluation of the use of

    saline over time is an example of _____ _____.

12. If you, as the nurse, questioned the wound care team's recommendations for a dressing for Harry George, you would be demonstrating the critical thinking attitude of

    _____ _____.

Exercise 2

 CD-ROM Activity

 45 minutes

 In this exercise you will visit Harry George, a 54-year old Caucasian male who was admitted to the hospital with symptoms of infection and swelling of the foot. Harry George has a history of abusing alcohol. He has been diagnosed with cellulitis and osteomyelitis of the foot. You may have worked with Harry George previously if you already completed Exercise 1 in this lesson or Lesson 16, 17 or 18.

   • Sign in to work at Pacific View Regional Hospital on the Medical-Surgical Floor for Period of Care 4. (*Note:* If you are already in the virtual hospital from a previous exercise, click on **Leave the Floor** and then **Restart the Program** to get to the sign-in window.)
   • Click on **Chart** and then on **401**. (*Remember:* You are not able to visit patients or administer medications during Period of Care 4. You are only able to review patients' records at this time.)
   • Click on and review the **Nursing Admission**.
   • Click on and review the **Nurse's Notes** from Wednesday 1200 to Wednesday 1900.
   • Next, click on **Consultations** and read the note from the Psychiatric Consult.
   • Finally, review the **Physician's Notes**.

1. Harry George has experienced the loss of his family and admits that his drinking problem has become serious. Critical thinking applied to assessment enables a nurse to develop a relevant plan of care. Complete the following critical thinking diagram for assessment of Harry George's situation by writing the letter of each of the critical thinking factors under its proper category.

Knowledge

1. _____

2. _____

3. _____

Experience   **Standards**

4. _____   **ASSESSMENT**   6. _____
                      SELF-CONCEPT

5. _____   7. _____

                      Attitudes

8. _____

9. _____

Critical Thinking Factors

a. Review the principles of self-concept.
b. Ask Harry George to discuss his relationship with his parents and its effects on his ability to cope with loss of his immediate family.
c. Apply principles of therapeutic communication in building a trusting relationship with Harry George.
d. Apply what you have learned from caring for patients with depression in the past to Harry George's case.
e. During your interview with Harry George, apply the criteria of phases of grief in determining the extent of his loss; take time to be thorough in your assessment.
f. When assessing Harry George's perception of self-concept, pay attention to his behavior and the content of his conversation.
g. Reflect on those situations when you have had to deal with agitated and restless patients.
h. Consider what you know about the symptoms and etiology of alcohol withdrawal.
i. Stay focused on the best interests of Harry George; keep him as comfortable as possible, managing his symptoms while attempting to assess his needs.

2. What are the five health dimensions for gathering a nursing health history?

3. When the nurse analyzes the data about Harry George's self-concept and family relation-ships, critical thinking ensures a complete database. Match each critical thinking standard below with its corresponding assessment approach.

Critical Thinking Standard

_____ Significant

_____ Consistent

_____ Accurate

Assessment Approach

a. During each encounter, observe the patient's facial expression and bodily movement.

b. Inquire "Mr. George, what does the loss of your family mean to you?"

c. Ask, "Mr. George, can you clarify for me exactly what happened before your wife decided to leave you?"

Applying the Nursing Process

👓 **Reading Assignment:** Nursing Process (Chapter 8)
Oxygenation (Chapter 29)

Patient: Patricia Newman, Medical-Surgical Floor, Room 406

Objectives:

- Assess the health care needs of patients in the case studies.
- Analyze data clusters from data gathered in a nursing assessment.
- Develop nursing diagnoses from data presented in the case studies.
- Identify the relationship of nursing diagnoses in a concept map.
- Identify priorities of nursing care for a case study patient.
- Develop goal and outcome statements.
- Discuss factors to consider in choosing nursing interventions.
- Identify types of nursing interventions.
- Evaluate the status of patients in the case studies.

Overview:

Each time you care for a patient, you apply the nursing process. The process begins with your assessment of a patient's health status. Analysis and interpretation of assessment data lead to the formation of nursing diagnoses and collaborative problems. After identifying relevant nursing diagnoses, you develop a plan of care. The plan directs how you implement the patient's care, using direct and indirect interventions. After administering interventions, you evaluate the patient's response and progress toward an improved level of health. The nursing process provides a framework to apply critical thinking skills in making competent decisions about the care of all patients.

Exercise 1

 CD-ROM Activity

 30 minutes

 In this exercise you will visit Patricia Newman, a 61-year-old Caucasian female who has a history of emphysema, osteoporosis, and hypertension. She has been admitted to the hospital in moderate respiratory distress. You may have worked with Patricia Newman previously if you already completed Lesson 3, 5, 9, or 10.

• Sign in to work at Pacific View Regional Hospital on the Medical-Surgical Floor for Period of Care 1. (*Note:* If you are already in the virtual hospital from a previous exercise, click on **Leave the Floor** and then **Restart the Program** to get to the sign-in window.)
• From the Patient List, select Patricia Newman (Room 406).
• Click on **Get Report**.
• Click on **Go to Nurses' Station**.
• Click on **Chart** and then on **406**.

1. Nursing assessment involves the careful review, analysis, and interpretation of data related to a patient's health status. Complete the following assessment flow sheet, based on your review of data for Patricia Newman in the following chart sections:

   • Nursing Admission
   • History and Physical

1. Vital signs and blood gases from 0700 clinical report	BP HR RR T SpO_2 pH PaO_2 HCO_3 $PaCO_2$
2. History of present illness	
3. Health promotion	Description of health: Usual BP: Flu shot: TB test: Routine self-exam:

4. Nutrition	Appetite: Meals/day:
	Fluid intake daily:
	Oral cavity:
	Other problems:
5. Respiratory	Cough:
	Lung sounds:
	Other symptoms:
6. Cardiovascular	Heart sounds:
	Abnormal findings:
7. Activity/Rest	Energy level:
	Other problems:

2. The patient's statement describing her health as "not very good" is an example of:
   a. objective data.
   b. back channeling.
   c. defining characteristic.
   d. subjective data.

 3. The measurement of objective data is based on accepted standards. For each of the following findings from Patricia Newman's assessment, identify the standard used in measurement. (*Study Tip:* Review page 112 in your textbook.)

Lung sounds

Temperature

Oral cavity

4. After reviewing the findings for Patricia Newman's cardiovascular and respiratory status, what other sources of similar data might you use? List two.

 • Click on **Return to Nurses' Station**.
  • Select room **406** at the bottom of the screen.
  • Review the **Initial Observations**.
  • Click on **Patient Care**.
  • Click on and review the examination findings for the **Chest** and then for the **Back & Spine**.

5. Data that you gather from a physical assessment help to confirm and broaden the data you have about potential problem areas. After reviewing assessment data on Patricia Newman, what problems are you beginning to identify? List three.

6. Data clusters are sets of signs or symptoms that are grouped together logically. Match each sign or symptom with its appropriate data cluster category.

Sign and Symptoms	**Data Cluster Category**
_____ Reduced energy level	a. Respiratory/oxygenation
_____ Dyspnea on exertion	b. Reduced energy level
_____ Productive cough	
_____ Oxygen saturation 92%	
_____ Feels "too tired to do much"	
_____ Requires frequent rest periods	
_____ Respirations labored	
_____ PaO$_2$ below normal	

7. As you identify clusters of data, you reason to recognize patterns or trends. Data often contain defining characteristics or criteria for nursing diagnoses. Listed below are several nursing diagnoses with defining characteristics. Which of these diagnoses apply to Patricia Newman? Select all that apply.

_____ Ineffective Airway Clearance: diminished breath sounds, dyspnea, adventitious breath sounds, ineffective cough, sputum production, changes in respiratory rate

_____ Impaired Gas Exchange: tachycardia, hypoxia, abnormal arterial blood gases, abnormal rate and depth of breathing, hypoxemia

_____ Ineffective Breathing Pattern: pursed-lip breathing, dyspnea, use of accessory muscles to breathe, respiratory rate higher than 24 per minute, altered chest excursion

_____ Ineffective Breathing Pattern: chronic obstructive pulmonary disorder

_____ Impaired Gas Exchange: emphysema

8. The related factors contributing to Patricia Newman's nursing diagnoses must be accurate for what reason?

9. Which of the following diagnostic statements apply to Patricia Newman? Select all that apply.

_____ Impaired Gas Exchange related to abnormal blood gas levels

_____ Activity Intolerance related to general weakness

_____ Imbalanced Nutrition: Less Than Body Requirements related to patient's need for high-protein diet

_____ Impaired Gas Exchange related to alveolar capillary changes

_____ Activity Intolerance related to insufficient exercise

_____ Imbalanced Nutrition: Less Than Body Requirements related to reduced intake of nutrients

10. Given Patricia Newman's numerous physical problems, develop a concept map by drawing arrows to show the association between nursing diagnoses. (*Study Tip:* Review pages 121 through 122 in your textbook.)

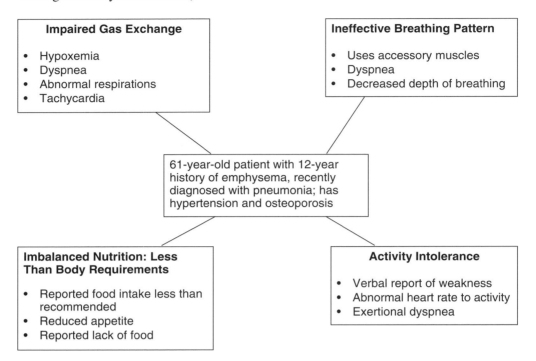

Impaired Gas Exchange

- Hypoxemia
- Dyspnea
- Abnormal respirations
- Tachycardia

Ineffective Breathing Pattern

- Uses accessory muscles
- Dyspnea
- Decreased depth of breathing

61-year-old patient with 12-year history of emphysema, recently diagnosed with pneumonia; has hypertension and osteoporosis

Imbalanced Nutrition: Less Than Body Requirements

- Reported food intake less than recommended
- Reduced appetite
- Reported lack of food

Activity Intolerance

- Verbal report of weakness
- Abnormal heart rate to activity
- Exertional dyspnea

Exercise 2

 CD-ROM Activity

 45 minutes

 In this exercise you will visit Patricia Newman, a 61-year-old Caucasian female who has a history of emphysema, osteoporosis, and hypertension. She has been admitted to the hospital in moderate respiratory distress. You may have worked with Patricia Newman previously if you already completed Exercise 1 of this lesson or Lessons 3, 5, 9, or 10.

- Sign in to work at Pacific View Regional Hospital on the Medical-Surgical Floor for Period of Care 2. (*Note:* If you are already in the virtual hospital from a previous exercise, click on **Leave the Floor** and then **Restart the Program** to get to the sign-in window.)
- From the Patient List, select Patricia Newman (Room 406).
- Click on **Get Report**.
- Click on **Go to Nurses' Station**.
- Click on **406** at the bottom of the screen to go to the patient's room.
- Review the **Initial Observations.**

1. As you review both the clinical report for 0730 to 1115 and the Initial Observations in the patient's room, you notice conflicting data. What would be your first action as you begin care for Patricia Newman?
   a. Discuss with her the plan of care for the day.
   b. Validate her pulmonary status by conducting a physical examination.
   c. Begin instruction on breathing exercises.
   d. Call the physician to review data from report.

• Click on **Patient Care**.

- Review the list of available assessment categories (yellow buttons), as well as the subcategories of each area (green buttons).

2. Because you want to validate Patricia Newman's pulmonary status, you will conduct a focused assessment. Which assessment categories should you include when examining Patricia Newman? Select all that apply.

_____   Sensory (Head & Neck)

_____   Lymphatic (Head & Neck)

_____   Musculoskeletal (Head & Neck)

_____   Neurologic (Head & Neck)

_____   Mental Status (Head & Neck)

_____   Integumentary (Chest)

_____   Cardiovascular (Chest)

_____   Respiratory (Chest)

_____   Musculoskeletal (Chest)

_____   Integumentary (Back & Spine)

_____   Musculoskeletal (Back & Spine)

_____   Respiratory (Back & Spine)

_____   Musculoskeletal (Abdomen)

_____   Gastrointestinal (Abdomen)

• Now complete your assessment of the patient based on your answer to question 2.

3. Earlier in Exercise 1, we identified the following nursing diagnoses for Patricia Newman: Impaired Gas Exchange, Ineffective Breathing Pattern, Activity Intolerance, and Imbalanced Nutrition: Less Than Body Requirements. Which of these diagnoses would be validated by your assessment in question 2?

• Click on **Nurse-Client Interactions**.

- Select and view the video titled **1100: Care Coordination**. (*Note:* Check the virtual clock to see whether enough time has elapsed. You can use the fast-forward feature to advance the time by 2-minute intervals if the video is not yet available. Then click again on **Patient Care** and **Nurse-Client Interactions** to refresh the screen.)
- Click on **Nurses' Station** at the bottom of the screen.
- Click on **Chart** and then on **406**.
- Review the **Physician's Notes**.

4. During the interaction the nurse collected valuable information from Patricia Newman, particularly since the physician has planned a number of consults. Listed below are two possible nursing diagnoses with defining characteristics that might apply to Patricia Newman. Which of the two do you believe is more appropriate for this patient?

    _____ Deficient Knowledge regarding appropriate diet (defining characteristics: verbalizes problem, inaccurate follow-through of instruction, inaccurate performance of test, inappropriate behavior)

    _____ Readiness for Enhanced Knowledge (defining characteristics: expresses an interest in learning, explains knowledge of topic, behaviors congruent with expressed knowledge, describes previous experience pertaining to topic)

5. Provide a rationale for the nursing diagnosis you chose in question 4.

 • While still in the chart, review the **History and Physical**.

6. For each of the two nursing diagnoses listed below, write a goal and two expected outcomes.

a. Impaired Gas Exchange

    Goal   Expected Outcomes

b. Readiness for Enhanced Knowledge

    Goal   Expected Outcomes

7. It is important to write goals and outcomes clearly. Explain what, if anything, is inaccurate about each of the outcome statements below.

   a. Respirations will be unlabored with a nonproductive cough:

   b. Patient's lung sounds will improve within 24 hours:

   c. Patient will feel less tired by discharge:

   d. Patient will become afebrile within 24 hours:

During the Nurse-Client Interaction video, the nurse suggested that the social worker might be able to assist with resources for smoking cessation programs and meal planning and preparation assistance for Patricia Newman. Fill in the blanks in the statements below that describe the process of consultation.

8. Consultation is based on the _____ _____ approach.

9. Consultation increases a nurse's _____ about a problem.

10. After a dietitian assesses Patricia Newman's knowledge of food sources and her ability to

    acquire food and prepare meals, the dietitian can more _____ identify the nutritional problem.

11. When making a consultation, it is important for the nurse not to _____ the consultant.

➡ • While still in the chart, review the **Physician's Orders**.

12. In developing a plan of care for Patricia Newman's diagnosis of Impaired Gas Exchange, the nurse selects a series of interventions. Match each intervention with its corresponding type. (*Study Tip:* To understand the rationale for the interventions, review textbook Chapter 29.)

Intervention	Type
_____ Administer oxygen at 2 L per nasal cannula.	a. Nurse-initiated
_____ Instruct patient on how to perform pursed-lip breathing.	b. Physician-initiated
_____ Position patient with head of bed elevated to 45 degrees.	c. Collaborative
_____ Administer bronchodilator by a metered-dose inhaler.	
_____ Have the patient perform cascade coughing every 1 hour.	
_____ Encourage oral fluids of 3 L daily.	

13. A nurse caring for Patricia Newman performs the following activities. Which activities are examples of indirect care measures? Select all that apply.

_____ Adjusts the oxygen flow meter to ensure that it runs correctly and checks condition of the tubing

_____ Coaches the patient on the technique for performing a cascade cough

_____ Documents the character of Patricia Newman's cough and her ability to expectorate mucus

_____ Consults with the respiratory therapist about the patient's use of a metered-dose inhaler

_____ Administers intravenous fluid infusion

14. For each of the expected outcomes listed below, write an evaluation measure.

a. Patient's lungs will clear without crackles within 48 hours

b. Patient's fluid intake will be 3 L every 24 hours

c. Patient will perform pursed-lip breathing correctly within 24 hours

d. Patient will experience less dyspnea while ambulating within 2 days

Exercise 3

 CD-ROM Activity

 30 minutes

 In this exercise you will visit Patricia Newman, a 61-year-old Caucasian female who has a history of emphysema, osteoporosis, and hypertension. She has been admitted to the hospital in moderate respiratory distress. You may have worked with Patricia Newman previously if you already completed Exercise 1 or 2 of this lesson or Lesson 3, 5, 9, or 10.

- Sign in to work at Pacific View Regional Hospital on the Medical-Surgical Floor for Period of Care 3. (*Note:* If you are already in the virtual hospital from a previous exercise, click on **Leave the Floor** and then **Restart the Program** to get to the sign-in window.)
- From the Patient List, select Patricia Newman (Room 406).
- Click on **Get Report**.

1. As you review the two clinical reports, complete the table below and evaluate the patient's clinical trend as either I (improving), S (remaining stable), or W (worsening).

Findings	0731-1115	1201-1500	Clinical Trend
SpO$_2$			
Blood pressure			
IV site			
Respiratory character			
Lung sounds			

2. Identify the evaluation measure used for each of Patricia Newman's physical findings listed below.

Finding	Evaluation Measure
Lungs less coarse	
IV site without redness	
SpO$_2$ 85%	
Respirations shallow	

3. If you already completed Exercise 1 of this lesson, you will remember that Patricia Newman had two nursing diagnoses for her respiratory problems. Those diagnoses are listed below, along with two outcomes that apply to each one.

   • Nursing diagnosis 1: Impaired Gas Exchange

   Outcomes: Patient will have a reduction in heart rate
   Patient will have an improved SpO$_2$

   • Nursing diagnosis 2: Ineffective Breathing Pattern

   Outcomes: Patient will report less breathlessness
   Respirations will be less labored

   Based on the clinical report findings you documented in questions 1 and 2, what would you do in regard to Patricia Newman's plan of care?

 • Click on **Go to Nurses' Station**.
   • Click on **Chart** and then on **406**.
   • Review the **Patient Education** file.
   • Review the **Consultations**.

4. Patricia Newman's teaching plan includes a number of different learning objectives, which are similar to expected outcomes. How would you, as the RN, measure the objective/outcome of "Patient will comply with dietary recommendations"?

Physical Examination and Vital Signs

∞ **Reading Assignment:** Vital Signs (Chapter 14)
Health Assessment and Physical Examination (Chapter 15)

Patients: Clarence Hughes, Medical-Surgical Floor, Room 404
Patricia Newman, Medical-Surgical Floor, Room 406

Objectives:

- Describe focused physical assessments required based on a patient's medical history findings.
- Recognize abnormal vital signs and physical assessment findings.
- Discuss techniques used to obtain accurate vital signs and physical assessment findings.
- Critique approaches used in the case studies for conducting a physical examination.
- Explain why certain physical examination techniques are used with patients in the case studies.
- Describe focused assessments relevant to changes in a patient's physical condition.
- Discuss how nursing therapies might change vital signs and physical examination findings.

Overview:

As a nurse, you are responsible for monitoring the condition and progress of your patients so that you can anticipate any clinical problems. Valuable sets of tools for assessing a patient's condition include conducting a physical examination and measuring vital signs. Findings from your assessment help to determine the patient's needs and nursing diagnoses and the types of interventions most appropriate. After you administer nursing interventions, physical examination and vital sign measurement also help you to evaluate how the patient responds and determine whether your interventions were successful. The exercises in this lesson will give you a clear idea of how physical examination and vital sign measurement become incorporated into a nurse's routine care and how approaches are individualized based on a patient's history and presenting clinical condition.

Exercise 1

 CD-ROM Activity

 45 minutes

In this exercise you will visit Clarence Hughes, a 73-year-old African-American male who was admitted to the hospital for a left total knee replacement. You will visit him on his third post-operative day. You may have worked with Clarence Hughes previously if you already completed Lesson 19.

- Sign in to work at Pacific View Regional Hospital on the Medical-Surgical Floor for Period of Care 1. (*Note:* If you are already in the virtual hospital from a previous exercise, click on **Leave the Floor** and then **Restart the Program** to get to the sign-in window.)
- From the Patient List, select Clarence Hughes (Room 404).
- Click on **Get Report**.
- Click on **Go to Nurses' Station**.
- Click on **Chart** and then on **404**.
- Click on and review the **History and Physical**.

1. Clarence Hughes' History and Physical summarizes the condition of his major body systems. For each of the history findings listed below, fill in the physical examination technique(s) you would use to further assess his condition.

History Findings	Physical Examination Techniques
Urinary stream less than it used to be	
Smoker for 50 years	
Receives pilocarpine drops	
Chronic pain in both knees	

2. The clinical report noted that Clarence Hughes feels constipated. List three physical examination techniques you might conduct to assess this problem area further.

3. Clarence Hughes' physical examination findings reveals a Glasgow Coma Scale (GCS) score of 15. This would be interpreted as:
   a. disoriented.
   b. unresponsive.
   c. normal.
   d. hyperactive.

4. Clarence Hughes' physical examination reveals normal S_1 and S_2 heart sounds. Indicate whether each of the following statements is true or false in regard to these findings.

   a. _____ S_1 represents the "dub" heard with the stethoscope.

   b. _____ S_2 represents the "dub" heard with the stethoscope.

   c. _____ There is a silent pause between S_1 and S_2.

   d. _____ Normally there is an irregular interval between each sequence of S_1 and S_2.

• Click on **Nurse's Notes**.
• Read the note for Wednesday 0715.

5. The nurse records the following about Clarence Hughes' knee: "may be slightly more swollen than yesterday." There are two approaches you could use to measure the extent of the edema more accurately. Describe each of these approaches. (*Study Tip:* See Figure 15-41 in your textbook.)

• Click on **Return to Nurses' Station**.
• Click on **404** at the bottom of the screen to enter Clarence Hughes' room.
• Review the **Initial Observations.**
• Click on **Patient Care** and then on **Physical Assessment**.
• Review the physical assessment findings for the following categories: **Head & Neck, Chest, Abdomen,** and **Lower Extremities**.

6. During the chest assessment, you observed a photo of the nurse assessing Clarence Hughes' cardiovascular function. At which site was the stethoscope placed to auscultate his heart rate?

7. Was the nurse using the correct portion of the stethoscope when assessing heart sounds? Give a rationale for your answer.

8. Clarence Hughes' cardiovascular assessment revealed that he had no murmurs, clicks, or rubs. Which portion of the stethoscope do you use to hear murmurs or other extra heart sounds?

9. The examination reveals "impaired sensation in the left leg." Which of the following correctly describe the techniques for assessing sensation? Select all that apply.

_____ Apply sharp end of a tongue blade to the skin as patient observes.

_____ Apply a light stimulus to the skin on both legs.

_____ Apply alternately, in a sporadic pattern, both a blunt and sharp end of a tongue blade.

_____ Apply sharp stimuli to areas with thicker skin.

_____ Apply a light stimulus to the skin as the patient closes the eyes.

10. Explain why the nurse was unable to palpate Clarence Hughes' popliteal pulse in the left leg. What would be another assessment option for the nurse to use?

11. Observe the techniques used by the nurse to examine the patient's abdomen for musculo-skeletal function. Was the nurse's technique in the photo correct? Give a rationale.

 • Now click on **Nurse-Client Interactions**.
 • Select and view the video titled **0730: Assessment/Perception of Care**. (*Note:* Check the virtual clock to see whether enough time has elapsed. You can use the fast-forward feature to advance the time by 2-minute intervals if the video is not yet available. Then click again on **Patient Care** and **Nurse-Client Interactions** to refresh the screen.)
 • Click on **Take Vital Signs**.

12. What factors at the present time would likely cause an increase in Clarence Hughes' heart rate? Select all that apply.

_____ Activity

_____ Pain

_____ Taking medication for constipation

_____ Sitting in bed with head elevated

13. If, when assessing a patient's radial pulse, the rate is irregular, you should count the rate for:
    a. 15 seconds.
    b. 30 seconds.
    c. 1 minute.
    d. 1 minute while another nurse takes an apical pulse.

Exercise 2

 CD-ROM Activity

 30 minutes

 In this exercise you will visit Clarence Hughes, a 73-year-old African-American male who was admitted to the hospital for a left total knee replacement. You will visit him on his third post-operative day. You may have worked with Clarence Hughes previously if you already completed Exercise 1 in this lesson or Lesson 19.

 • Sign in to work at Pacific View Regional Hospital on the Medical-Surgical Floor for Period of Care 2. (*Note:* If you are already in the virtual hospital from a previous exercise, click on **Leave the Floor** and then **Restart the Program** to get to the sign-in window.)
 • From the Patient List, select Clarence Hughes (Room 404).

- Click on **Get Report**.
- Click on **Go to Nurses' Station**.
- Click on **EPR** and **Login**.
- Select **404** from the Patient drop-down menu and **Vital Signs** from the Category drop-down menu.

1. In the flow chart below, enter Clarence Hughes' vital signs for the designated time periods.

Result	BP	HR	RR	SpO$_2$
Tuesday 1600				
Tuesday 2300				
Wednesday 0715				

2. At this point in time, after reviewing your flow chart, Clarence Hughes' condition can best be described as:
   a. normal and stable.
   b. bradycardic with normal BP, respirations, and oxygen saturation.
   c. hypotensive and bradycardic with normal respirations and oxygen saturation.
   d. low oxygen saturation with hypotension, normal heart rate, and respirations.

3. Pulse oximetry is a reliable, indirect measure of oxygen saturation. Indicate whether each of the following descriptions of factors affecting oxygen saturation is true or false.

   a. _____   Oxygen saturation would be lowered by an obstruction in the pulmonary capillaries.

   b. _____   Oxygen saturation would be lowered by a reduction in hemoglobin.

   c. _____   Oxygen saturation would be lowered by build-up of edema between the alveoli and pulmonary capillaries.

   d. _____   Oxygen saturation would be lowered by a transfusion of red blood cells.

- Click on **Exit EPR**.
- Select **404** at the bottom of the screen.
- Review the **Initial Observations.**
- Click on **Patient Care** and then **Nurse-Client Interactions**.
- Select and view the video titled **1115: Intervention—Airway**. (*Note:* Check the virtual clock to see whether enough time has elapsed. You can use the fast-forward feature to advance the time by 2-minute intervals if the video is not yet available. Then click again on **Patient Care** and **Nurse-Client Interactions** to refresh the screen.)
- Click on **Take Vital Signs** at the top of the screen.

4. Clarence Hughes is obviously in acute distress. Enter his 1115 vital sign results in the bottom row of the chart below. Then, for comparison purposes, enter his vital signs for the three earlier times listed. (*Note:* You can find these results in the EPR, or you can copy your answers from question 1 of this exercise.)

Result	BP	HR	RR	SpO$_2$
Tuesday 1600				
Tuesday 2300				
Wednesday 0715				
Wednesday 1115				

5. Below, explain the clinical changes occurring for each of Clarence Hughes' vital signs listed in the table above.

   a. Change in BP:

   b. Change in heart rate:

   c. Change in respirations:

   d. Change in SpO$_2$:

6. In measuring vital signs it is important to be accurate. Which of the following factors could cause a false high value in Clarence Hughes' blood pressure? Select all that apply.

   _____ Loose-fitting cuff

   _____ BP cuff too wide

   _____ BP cuff inflated too slowly

   _____ Patient's arm above heart level

   _____ BP cuff deflated too quickly

7. You are the nurse preparing to examine Clarence Hughes. Of the following list of examination categories, which would you identify as priority assessments for this patient? Select all that apply.

_____ Sensory (Head & Neck)

_____ Mental Status (Head & Neck)

_____ Thyroid (Head & Neck)

_____ Respiratory (Chest)

_____ Cardiovascular (Chest)

_____ Integumentary (Chest)

_____ Integumentary (Upper Extremities)

_____ Vascular (Upper Extremities)

_____ Gastrointestinal (Abdomen)

_____ Musculoskeletal (Abdomen)

_____ Vascular (Lower Extremities)

_____ Integumentary (Lower Extremities)

→ • Now, click on **Patient Care** and then on **Physical Assessment**.
 • Review the physical assessment findings for the following categories: **Head & Neck (Mental Status)**, **Upper Extremities** (**Integumentary** and **Vascular**), **Chest**, and **Lower Extremities**.

8. Consider what you observed in the video interaction and physical assessment. Match each of the findings below with its likely cause.

Findings	**Cause**
_____ Altered peripheral circulation	a. Reduced oxygen to brain
_____ Patient sitting up	b. Pulmonary condition affecting oxygenation
_____ Tachypnea	c. Attempt to improve ventilation
_____ Anxious and agitated	d. Color in lower extremities pale

→ • Click on **Chart** and then click on **404**.
 • Review the **Physician's Orders**.

9. Explain why the physician ordered an arterial blood gas (ABG).

For questions 10 through 15, fill in the blanks with the appropriate terms describing pulse oximetry.

10. The _____ or _____ is an appropriate site for place-ment of a spring-loaded oximeter probe.

11. Removal of _____ is necessary to ensure proper light transmission when using an oximeter.

12. The pulse wave on the oximeter will be _____ by peripheral edema.

13. Normally, when first applying an oximeter probe, it takes _____ to _____ seconds for a reading to appear.

→ • Click on **Return to Room 404**.
   • Click on **Leave the Floor** and then **Restart the Program**.
   • Sign in to work at Pacific View Regional Hospital on the Medical-Surgical Floor for Period of Care 3.
   • From the Patient List, select Clarence Hughes (Room 404).
   • Click on **Get Report**.
   • Review the clinical report.
   • Click on **Go to Nurses' Station**.

14. Clarence Hughes was experiencing a pulmonary embolus. An embolus blocks blood flow in an artery supplying blood to the lung. In this case, the embolus probably originated in the patient's popliteal vein, where tests have shown a thrombus is located. Which of the follow-ing are signs of venous insufficiency? Select all that apply.

_____   Absent pulse

_____   Marked edema

_____   Cyanosis of the skin

_____   Normal pulse

_____   Shiny skin

Exercise 3

 CD-ROM Activity

 30 minutes

 Patricia Newman is a 61-year-old Caucasian female with a history of emphysema for 12 years. She has been admitted to the emergency department in moderate respiratory distress. You may have worked with Patricia Newman previously if you already completed Lesson 2, 5, 9, or 10.

- Sign in to work at Pacific View Regional Hospital on the Medical-Surgical Floor for Period of Care 1. (*Note:* If you are already in the virtual hospital from a previous exercise, click on **Leave the Floor** and then **Restart the Program** to get to the sign-in window.)
- From the Patient List, select Patricia Newman (Room 406).
- Click on **Get Report**.

1. Match each of the vital sign findings on the left with its corresponding terminology on the right.

Vital Sign Finding	Term
_____ 168/94	a. Tachypneic
_____ 112	b. Hypertensive
_____ 32	c. Febrile
_____ 102° F	d. Tachycardic

- Click on **Go to Nurses' Station**.
- Click on **Chart** and then on **406**.
- Click on and review the **History and Physical**.

2. Patricia Newman has a history of emphysema and hypertension. What is one factor in her history that could be associated with both conditions?

3. Patricia Newman's physical examination reveals coarse crackles throughout the lung fields. Which of the entries below correctly describe the features of crackles? Select all that apply.

_____ Heard over anterior lateral lung field

_____ Best heard in dependent lobes

_____ Primarily heard over trachea and bronchi

_____ Caused by high-velocity air flow

_____ Result of inflamed pleura

_____ Result of sudden reinflation of alveoli

_____ High-pitched, fine, and short sound

_____ Dry, grating sound

_____ Low-pitched, rumbling sound

 • Click on **Return to Nurses' Station**.
   • Click on **406** at the bottom of the screen to go to Patricia Newman's room.
   • Review the **Initial Observations.**
   • Click on **Patient Care** and then **Nurse-Client Interactions**.
   • Select and view the video titled **0730: Prioritizing Interventions**. (*Note:* Check the virtual clock to see whether enough time has elapsed. You can use the fast-forward feature to advance the time by 2-minute intervals if the video is not yet available. Then click again on **Patient Care** and **Nurse-Client Interactions** to refresh the screen.)
   • Now click on **Physical Assessment**.
   • Click on **Chest** and observe the complete examination of the chest.

4. The respiratory assessment of the chest notes that Patricia Newman's breathing is labored and shallow. What assessment techniques are used to determine these findings?

5. Again, observe the nurse as she performs the respiratory assessment of the chest. Where was the stethoscope placed by the nurse? What should be the next five placements of the stethoscope if the nurse is assessing anteriorly?

• Now click on **Back & Spine** and then on **Respiratory**.

6. Observe the respiratory assessment findings for the back and spine. The findings note that Patricia Newman has hyperesonance to percussion. Explain the reason for this finding.

➡ • Click on **Take Vital Signs** at the top of the screen.

7. Match each blood pressure type with its corresponding auscultatory sound.

Blood Pressure Type	**Auscultatory Sound**
_____ Systolic pressure	a. First Korotkoff sound
_____ Diastolic pressure	b. Second Korotkoff sound
	c. Third Korotkoff sound
	d. Fourth Korotkoff sound
	e. Fifth Korotkoff sound

8. Because Patricia Newman is hypertensive, she is at risk for presenting an auscultatory gap during blood pressure measurement.

   a. What is an auscultatory gap?

   b. The gap typically occurs between which heart sounds?

   c. How do you avoid an auscultatory gap when measuring BP?

Communication with the Patient and the Health Care Team

📖 **Reading Assignment:** Communication (Chapter 10)

Patients: Dorothy Grant, Obstetrics Floor, Room 201
Kathryn Doyle, Skilled Nursing Floor, Room 503

Objectives:

- Discuss perceptions of communication interactions viewed in the case studies.
- Describe levels of communication.
- Identify forms of communication viewed in the case studies.
- Describe elements of professional communication.
- Identify factors that create barriers to communication.
- Identify therapeutic communication techniques.

Overview:

At the core of nursing are the caring relationships formed between nurses and patients. All of our behavior communicates, and all communication influences the behavior of others. Communication is the means for establishing therapeutic relationships with patients. The ability to communicate effectively helps you to establish the important connection that allows you to deliver quality care to patients.

Talking *with* patients, not *at* patients, can be difficult. The same is true in regard to patients' families. Communication requires sensitivity, active participation, and an astute interpretation of what people convey through their words and behavior. You must be willing to know a patient and to reveal a bit of yourself in order to establish the trust and confidence necessary to communicate therapeutically.

Exercise 1

 CD-ROM Activity

 45 minutes

In this exercise you will visit Dorothy Grant, a pregnant 25-year-old who was admitted to the hospital after blunt trauma to the abdomen. You may have worked with Dorothy Grant previously if you already completed Lesson 18.

- Sign in to work at Pacific View Regional Hospital on the Obstetrics Floor for Period of Care 2. (*Note:* If you are already in the virtual hospital from a previous exercise, click on **Leave the Floor** and then **Restart the Program** to get to the sign-in window.)
- From the Patient List, select Dorothy Grant (Room 201).
- Click on **Get Report**.
- Click on **Go to Nurses' Station**.
- Click on **Chart** and then on **201**.
- Click on and review the **Nursing Admission**.

1. The report tells you that the patient has been anxious and crying. As you prepare to go to Dorothy Grant's room to meet her, what might you consider doing in your initial communication approach? Describe in detail.

2. Active listening will be an important communication technique as you talk with Dorothy Grant. Several nonverbal skills that facilitate attentive listening can be remembered by the acronym SOLER. Describe each of these skills below.

    S

    O

    L

    E

    R

 - Click on **Return to Nurses' Station**.
- Click on **201** at bottom of screen.
- Review the **Initial Observations**.
- Click on **Patient Care** and then **Nurse-Client Interactions**.
- Select and view the video titled **1115: Nurse-Patient Communication**. (*Note:* Check the virtual clock to see whether enough time has elapsed. You can use the fast-forward feature to advance the time by 2-minute intervals if the video is not yet available. Then click again on **Patient Care** and **Nurse-Client Interactions** to refresh the screen.)

3. The nurse opens the conversation by asking, "Would you like to talk about your concerns?"

   a. What type of question is this?

   b. Was this the most appropriate way to begin the conversation? If not, how would you restate the question?

→ • Observe the video interaction again.

4. As you observe the nurse interact with Dorothy Grant, identify which of the following listening techniques the nurse uses. Select all that apply.

   _____   Sit facing patient

   _____   Observe an open posture

   _____   Lean toward patient

   _____   Establish/maintain eye contact

   _____   Relax

5. During the video, the nurse says to the patient, "Right now, your first priority is your well-being and the well-being of your baby." This is an example of what therapeutic technique?
   a. Empathy
   b. Sharing hope
   c. Providing information
   d. Paraphrasing

6. Dorothy Grant expresses how valuable her sister has been as a resource, but she states that her parents "act like nothing is going on."

   a. The nurse responds, "That must be so frustrating." What type of communication technique is this?

   b. What is the patient's response to this technique?

7. What communication and caring technique does the nurse use to initially focus on the importance of monitoring Dorothy Grant's obstetric condition? What is the purpose of this technique?

➤ • Observe the video interaction one final time.

8. Complete the categories listed below and describe Dorothy Grant's nonverbal behaviors for each category.

Personal appearance

Facial expression

Eye contact

Gestures

Sounds

9. As the nurse interacts with Dorothy Grant, she is assuming which zone of personal space?
   a. Public zone
   b. Personal zone
   c. Intimate zone
   d. Social zone

Exercise 2

 CD-ROM Activity

 30 minutes

 In this exercise you will visit Kathryn Doyle, a 79-year-old Caucasian female who was admitted following a fall at home in which she sustained a left hip fracture. You may have worked with Kathryn Doyle previously if you already completed Lesson 6, 7, or 8.

- Sign in to work at Pacific View Regional Hospital on the Skilled Nursing Floor for Period of Care 1. (*Note:* If you are already in the virtual hospital from a previous exercise, click on **Leave the Floor** and then **Restart the Program** to get to the sign-in window.)
- From the Patient List, select Kathryn Doyle (Room 503).
- Click on **Get Report**.
- Click on **Go to Nurses' Station**.
- Click on **Chart** and then on **503**.
- Review the patient's **History and Physical**.
- Next, review the **Nursing Admission**, paying particular attention to the Self-Perception and Role Relationships sections.
- Click on **Return to Nurses' Station**.
- Click on Room **503** at the bottom of the screen.
- Review the **Initial Observations**.
- Click on **Patient Care** and then **Nurse-Client Interactions**.
- Select and view the video titled **0730: Assessment—Biopsychosocial**. (*Note:* Check the virtual clock to see whether enough time has elapsed. You can use the fast-forward feature to advance the time by 2-minute intervals if the video is not yet available. Then click again on **Patient Care** and **Nurse-Client Interactions** to refresh the screen.)

  1. After reviewing data from the History and Physical and Nursing Admission, you know that Kathryn Doyle has concerns about returning home. In the video interaction between the nurse and patient, what nonverbal behavior did Kathryn Doyle display in each of the following categories?

Voice tone

Facial expression

Eye contact

2. List three characteristics of eye contact.

→ • Observe the same video once again.

3. Kathryn Doyle stated, "I just don't feel like myself." The nurse responded, "Do you have any concerns you would like to talk about?" Was the nurse's response appropriate? Explain.

4. Kathryn Doyle explains, "Well, I've been thinking of going home and wondering just what it's going to be like." For each of the communication techniques listed below, write an appropriate response to learn more about her feelings toward going home.

Paraphrasing

Sharing observation

Clarifying

→ • Now, select and view the video titled **0733: Planning—Fact Finding**. (*Note:* Check the virtual clock to see whether enough time has elapsed. You can use the fast-forward feature to advance the time by 2-minute intervals if the video is not yet available. Then click again on **Patient Care** and **Nurse-Client Interactions** to refresh the screen.)

5. The nurse responds, "Oh, why do you think that is?" What type of response is this?
   a. Asking for explanation
   b. Clarifying
   c. Focusing
   d. Automatic response

6. What would have been a better response on the part of the nurse?

7. Listed below are some nontherapeutic communication techniques. Match each type with its corresponding example.

**Nontherapeutic e
Communication Technique**

_____ Automatic response

_____ False reassurance

_____ Disapproval

_____ Sympathy

Example

a. "You shouldn't stop eating. It will make it difficult for your hip to heal."

b. "Sons just do not understand their mothers."

c. "Don't be concerned. Your weight loss is not a problem."

d. "I'm sorry about your husband. It must be such a heavy burden for you."

8. List five principles needed for professional communication.

9. By using assertive behavior, a nurse has the advantage of conveying the ability to:
   a. empathize.
   b. make decisions.
   c. judge others' behavior.
   d. depend on others for agreement.

Patient Education in Practice

/OO **Reading Assignment:** Patient Education (Chapter 11)
Administering Medications (Chapter 16)

Patient: Patricia Newman, Medical-Surgical Floor, Room 406

Objectives:

- Identify purposes of patient education.
- Describe basic learning principles.
- Assess the learning needs of a case study patient.
- Apply critical thinking in planning a teaching plan for a case study patient.
- Describe domains of learning to include in a patient's plan of care.
- Discuss factors to consider in designing a teaching plan.
- Identify factors that influence a patient's readiness to learn.
- Write learning objectives for a teaching plan.
- Discuss teaching methods appropriate to selected case study patients.
- Identify approaches for evaluating learning.

Overview:

It is your responsibility as a nurse to provide patient education so that patients and families are able to make informed decisions about their health and to assume self-care activities. Patient education is one of your most important roles as a nurse. Your challenge is to develop the best teaching plan that matches the patient's learning needs and ability to learn with relevant and appropriate teaching strategies. Because most patients continue health care activities in the home, you must be aware of all of the educational resources available to ensure a smooth and safe transition of care. Evaluation of patient learning is also critical to ensure that patients have obtained necessary knowledge and the ability to perform self-care activities.

Exercise 1

 CD-ROM Activity

 45 minutes

 In this exercise you will visit Patricia Newman, a 61-year-old Caucasian female who has a history of emphysema, osteoporosis, and hypertension. She has been admitted to the hospital in moderate respiratory distress. You may have worked with Patricia Newman previously if you already completed Lesson 2, 3, 9, or 10.

- Sign in to work at Pacific View Regional Hospital on the Medical-Surgical Floor for Period of Care 1. (*Note:* If you are already in the virtual hospital from a previous exercise, click on **Leave the Floor** and then **Restart the Program** to get to the sign-in window.)
- From the Patient List, select Patricia Newman (Room 406).
- Click on **Get Report**.
- Click on **Go to Nurses' Station**.
- Click on **Chart** and then on **406**.
- Review the **Nursing Admission**.

1. Using data from the Nursing Admission, consider each of the following learning principles and describe how they apply to Patricia Newman. Be specific.

Attention set

Compliance

Psychosocial adaptation to illness

Physical capability

2. What behavior increases Patricia Newman's risk for worsening emphysema?
   a. Not getting a flu shot
   b. Family history of lung disease
   c. Smoking cigarettes
   d. Becoming underweight

 • Still in the chart, click and review the **Physician's Orders**.
   • Now click on **Return to Nurses' Station**; then click on the **Drug** icon at the bottom of the screen and review all of the medications ordered for Patricia Newman (*Study Tip:* You may also use your Pharmacology textbook to review Patricia Newman's ordered medications.)
   • Click on **Return to Nurses' Station**.
   • Click on **Chart** then on **406**.
   • Click on **Consultations** and review the consult notes.

3. Based on the information you have reviewed so far, list four learning needs that apply to Patricia Newman.

4. Consider Patricia Newman's learning needs. Below, match each learning need with its corresponding learning domain.

Learning Need	**Learning Domain**
_____ Adopting health promotion behaviors (e.g., routine breast self-exams)	a. Cognitive
	b. Affective
_____ Understanding the benefits achieved from not smoking	c. Psychomotor
_____ Manipulation of a metered-dose inhaler	
_____ Being able to count caloric intake each day	

 • Click on **Return to Nurses' Station**.
   • Click on **406** at the bottom of the screen.
   • Review the **Initial Observations.**
   • Click on **Patient Care** and then on **Nurse-Client Interactions**.
   • Select and view the videos titled **0730: Prioritizing Interventions** and **0740: Evaluation— Response to Care**. (*Note:* Check the virtual clock to see whether enough time has elapsed. You can use the fast-forward feature to advance the time by 2-minute intervals if the video is not yet available. Then click again on **Patient Care** and **Nurse-Client Interactions** to refresh the screen.)

5. The respiratory therapist will be working with Patricia Newman on use of a peak flow meter as a means to detect changes in her airway resistance. Which of the following factors should be assessed in relation to Patricia Newman's ability to learn? Select all that apply.

_____ Distractors in the room during demonstration of meter

_____ Coordination and endurance to hold meter and perform breathing maneuver

_____ Patient's belief in need to improve lung function

_____ Patient's learning style preference

6. As Patricia Newman's nurse, you identify the nursing diagnosis of Deficient Knowledge regarding use of peak flow meter related to lack of exposure to information. You collaborate with the respiratory therapist to develop a teaching plan for Patricia Newman so that she can use the meter routinely at home. Complete the following critical thinking diagram for planning by writing the letter of each critical thinking factor under its proper category.

Knowledge

1. _____

2. _____

Experience   **PLANNING**   **Standards**

3. _____   4. _____

5. _____

Attitudes

6. _____

Critical Thinking Factors

a. Be creative in planning to have neighbor attend teaching session so that patient will have a coach to reinforce meter technique.
b. Review information regarding the effects emphysema has on peak flow rate.
c. Consider how you have instructed patients in the past on use of medical devices.
d. Review manufacturer's directions for proper use of flow meter.
e. Individualize teaching sessions to plan for frequent rest periods and reinforcement.
f. Consider learning principles that influence patient's motivation.

7. Write a learning objective for teaching Patricia Newman on the use of a peak flow meter.

• Click on **Chart** and then on **406**.
• Review the **Patient Education** file.

8. For each of the learning goals listed on Patricia Newman's teaching plan, critique and explain how the goal or objective should be written more clearly.

a. Patient will comply with dietary recommendations:

b. Patient will understand rationale and perform pursed-lip breathing:

c. Patient will demonstrate correct use of MDI:

9. When instructing Patricia Newman on the use of the peak flow meter, the nurse should combine demonstration with discussion. What might you include in the discussion?

 • Click on **Return to Room 406**.
• Click on **Patient Care** and then on **Nurse-Client Interactions**.
• Select and view the video titled **0750: Evaluation—Patient Teaching**. (*Note:* Check the virtual clock to see whether enough time has elapsed. You can use the fast-forward feature to advance the time by 2-minute intervals if the video is not yet available. Then click again on **Patient Care** and **Nurse-Client Interactions** to refresh the screen.)

10. During the interaction, the nurse missed an opportunity to evaluate Patricia Newman's learning. What should the nurse have done?

Exercise 2

 CD-ROM Activity

 30 minutes

 In this exercise you will visit Patricia Newman, a 61-year-old Caucasian female who has a history of emphysema, osteoporosis, and hypertension. She has been admitted to the hospital in moderate respiratory distress. You may have worked with Patricia Newman previously if you already completed Exercise 1 of this lesson or Lesson 2, 3, 9, or 10.

- Sign in to work at Pacific View Regional Hospital on the Medical-Surgical Floor for Period of Care 2. (*Note:* If you are already in the virtual hospital from a previous exercise, click on **Leave the Floor** and then **Restart the Program** to get to the sign-in window.)
- From the Patient List, select Patricia Newman (Room 406).
- Click on **Get Report**.
- Click on **Go to Nurses' Station**.
- Click on **Chart** and then on **406**.
- Review the **Nursing Admission**.
- Review the **Physician's Orders**.

1. There are three primary purposes of patient education. Match each education topic listed below with the purpose applicable to Patricia Newman.

Education Topic	Purpose
_____ Walking more frequently at longer intervals	a. Health promotion
_____ Quitting smoking	b. Health restoration
_____ Purpose and schedule of inhaler	c. Coping with impaired function
_____ Purpose of flu shots	
_____ Administration of home oxygen	

 - Click on **Return to Nurses' Station**.
- Select Room **406** at the bottom of the screen to go to the patient's room.
- Review the **Initial Observations.**
- Click on **Patient Care** and then on **Nurse-Client Interactions**.
- Select and view the video titled **1100: Care Coordination**. (*Note:* Check the virtual clock to see whether enough time has elapsed. You can use the fast-forward feature to advance the time by 2-minute intervals if the video is not yet available. Then click again on **Patient Care** and **Nurse-Client Interactions** to refresh the screen.)

2. Patricia Newman's statement "I know I should quit smoking" is an example of which learning principle?
   a. Ability to learn
   b. A learning need
   c. Motivation
   d. Compliance

3. Indicate which of the following statements is true or false.

a. _____ Patients who are highly anxious will often be motivated to learn.

b. _____ Patients learn better when you build on their existing level of knowledge.

c. _____ Patients who are in pain often have an impaired ability to learn.

d. _____ Assessing whether a patient is able to convert food portions to calories and add total calories determines an ability to learn.

e. _____ A patient who grieves over the loss of physical function will most likely learn about long-range health restrictions during the phase of bargaining.

 4. The physician ordered Patricia Newman to self-administer ipratropium bromide by metered-dose inhaler. Based on her admission data, what aspect of this activity might be difficult for the patient to perform? (*Study Tip:* Review pages 439 through 443 in your textbook.)
   a. Reading the medication label
   b. Understanding the directions
   c. Depressing the medication canister
   d. Sitting up to inhale the medication

 • Click on **Chart** and then on **406**.
   • Review the **Patient Education** file.

5. Patricia Newman will be receiving instruction on a number of topics. Match each teaching topic with its appropriate instructional method.

Instructional Method	**Teaching Topic**
_____ Simulation	a. Pursed-lip breathing
_____ Demonstration	b. Side effects of medications
_____ Role playing	c. Planning a dinner high in protein
_____ One-to-one discussion	d. Learning to say no when a friend offers a cigarette
_____ Use of analogies	e. Explaining how high blood pressure creates an effect similar to forcing water through a constricted hose

6. For each of the instructional topics listed below, identify the correct evaluation method.

Self-administration of a metered-dose inhaler

Patient's ability to increase distance walking

Patient's compliance with a high-caloric diet

Documentation Principles

∞ **Reading Assignment:** Informatics and Documentation (Chapter 9)

Patients: Kathryn Doyle, Skilled Nursing Floor, Room 503
Pablo Rodriguez, Medical-Surgical Floor, Room 405

Objectives:

- Identify the purpose of medical records.
- Identify elements of quality documentation in written records and verbal reports.
- Apply use of military time in recording.
- Write a nursing progress note.
- Explain the purpose of flow charting.
- Critique the quality of a change-of-shift report.
- Describe elements of a telephone order.
- Explain the type of information to communicate when a patient's condition changes.

Overview:

Recording and reporting are two nursing skills that must be performed accurately and in a timely and effective manner. The quality of your nursing care depends on your ability to communicate with other nurses and members of the health care team. All health care providers must know their patients, the problems they develop, their progress, and their response to treatments. Excellent documentation and reporting of information ensures that you have the knowledge you need about patients to provide continuity of care from shift to shift or visit to visit. In order for you to become competent in documentation, you must follow both legal and regulatory standards for how and what to record about your patients' care.

Exercise 1

 CD-ROM Activity

 45 minutes

 In this exercise you will visit Kathryn Doyle, a 79-year-old Caucasian female who entered the skilled nursing unit after repair of an intertrochanteric fracture 2 weeks ago. You may have worked with Kathryn Doyle previously if you already completed Lesson 4, 7, or 8.

- Sign in to work at Pacific View Regional Hospital on the Skilled Nursing Floor for Period of Care 1. (*Note:* If you are already in the virtual hospital from a previous exercise, click on **Leave the Floor** and then **Restart the Program** to get to the sign-in window.)
- From the Patient List, select Kathryn Doyle (Room 503).
- Click on **Get Report**.

1. After reviewing the report summary, list two examples of incomplete or inaccurate information given in the report.

2. The report summary notes that Kathryn Doyle received oxycodone and acetaminophen for pain in the left hip. What criteria should have been included in the description of the patient's pain? Select all that apply.

   _____ Condition of right hip

   _____ Onset of pain

   _____ Severity of pain

   _____ Action of pain medication

   _____ Factors that worsen pain

   _____ Duration of pain

 - Click on **Go to Nurses' Station**.
- Click on **Chart** and then on **503**.
- Click on **Nurse's Notes** and review the note for Wednesday 0715.
- Now, click on **Return to Nurses' Station**.
- Click on **EPR** and then **Login**.
- Select **503** from the Patient drop-down menu and choose **Vital Signs** from the Category drop-down menu.

3. Although the nurse's note reported that Kathryn Doyle had a low-grade fever, more accurate information was available in the EPR. What was Kathryn Doyle's actual temperature?

 • Review the other entries on the Vital Signs flow sheet.

4. List two advantages of a flow sheet.

 • Click on **Exit EPR**.
   • Click on **Chart** and then on **503**.
   • Click on **Nurse's Notes** and review the note for Wednesday 0555.

5. The entry of 0555 represents what time in standard time notation?
   a. 5:55 p.m.
   b. 12:05 a.m.
   c. 5:55 a.m.
   d. 12:55 p.m.

6. When updating the Kardex, the nurse should include which of the following? Select all that apply.

   _____ Contact number for the next of kin

   _____ The priority nursing diagnosis

   _____ Planned tests and procedures

   _____ Patient's response to analgesics

   _____ Medical diagnosis

7. The nurse's entry, "States she 'could not get comfortable,'" is an example of which documentation characteristic?
   a. Accuracy
   b. Complete
   c. Factual
   d. Current

8. Rewrite the nurse's note for Wednesday 0555 using the PIE format below.

   P

   I

   E

9. How might the nurse have made the Wednesday 0555 nurse's note more complete in regard to Kathryn Doyle's problem of pain management?

→ • Still in the chart, review the **Nurse's Notes** for Tuesday at 1825.
  • Next, go to the **Physician's Orders** and review the entry for Tuesday at 1530.

10. The nurse's note for 1825 refers to a TO verified.

    a. Does the nurse's signature on this note verify the telephone order?

    b. Is the nurse's signature the correct way for signing off a note? If not, explain.

    c. Are nurses required to have a witness listen in on all telephone orders?

11. Is the physician's order for the psychiatric consult completed correctly? Explain.

• Click on **Nursing Admission** and review the summary.

12. Medical records serve several purposes. Below, match each application of information from Kathryn Doyle's record with its purpose.

Application	**Purpose**
_____ Data show that Kathryn Doyle's allergy history was entered.	a. Communication of patient problem
_____ A review of Kathryn Doyle's self-perception helps demonstrate factors that influence a person's body image.	b. Use of records to research characteristics of patients who have hip surgery
_____ Kathryn Doyle's assessment shows she is sleeping poorly, tires easily, and receives no regular exercise.	c. Auditing of chart for regulatory requirements
_____ Kathryn Doyle is age 79. She has a history of osteoporosis, she fell at home, and she takes calcium daily.	d. Education for understanding nature of nursing concepts

Exercise 2

 CD-ROM Activity

 30 minutes

In this exercise you will visit Pablo Rodriguez, a 71-year-old Hispanic male who is suffering from advanced non-small cell lung carcinoma. You may have worked with Pablo Rodriguez previously if you already completed Lesson 11, 12, 13, or 19.

• Sign in to work at Pacific View Regional Hospital on the Medical-Surgical Floor for Period of Care 1. (*Note:* If you are already in the virtual hospital from a previous exercise, click on **Leave the Floor** and then **Restart the Program** to get to the sign-in window.)
• From the Patient List, select Pablo Rodriguez (Room 405).
• Click on **Get Report**.

1. The report summary is an example of the information typically shared between nurses during a change-of-shift report. One of the advantages of oral reports is the ability to ask questions. After reviewing Pablo Rodriguez's report, list three questions you might ask the night nurse.

2. Indicate whether each of the following statements is true or false.

a. _____ When you are giving a report, it is most important to be complete, so take whatever time is needed.

b. _____ One of the best methods of report is to read information from the patient's Kardex.

c. _____ When giving a transfer report, you should include a discussion of any assessments that should be completed shortly after the transfer.

d. _____ Whenever you take a telephone report, you should repeat the entire report to ensure accuracy.

e. _____ Telephone orders and verbal orders need to be cosigned by the ordering physician, usually within 24 hours.

3. Which of the following is a chief advantage of a taped shift report?
   a. Allows report to be completed in an efficient, timely manner
   b. Reduces errors with false reporting
   c. Increases the amount of information provided between the shifts
   d. Provides a forum for the nurse to report family concerns

4. For each action listed below, write *Do* if the action correctly applies to the change-of-shift report or write *Don't* if it does not apply to the change-of-shift report. For *Don't* answers, explain your reasoning.

   a. Describe the basic steps of how the patient uses a PCA.

   b. Describe objective measures such as "oxygen at 3 liters."

   c. Evaluate result of morphine when given for pain in nodules.

   d. Review the patient's age, occupation, and education.

   e. Identify and explain the patient's immediate priorities of care.

 • Click on **Go to Nurses' Station**.
   • Click on **405** at the bottom of the screen to go to the patient's room.
   • Review the **Initial Observations.**
   • Click on **Patient Care** and then **Nurse-Client Interactions**.
   • Select and view the video titled **0735: Patient Perceptions**. (*Note:* Check the virtual clock to see whether enough time has elapsed. You can use the fast-forward feature to advance the time by 2-minute intervals if the video is not yet available. Then click again on **Patient Care** and **Nurse-Client Interactions** to refresh the screen.)

5. Observe and listen to the video several times. Now pretend you are the nurse in the video and write a DAR note below that describes the interaction with Pablo Rodriguez.

D

A

R

➔ • Click on **Chart** and then on **405**.
  • Read the **Nurse's Notes**.

6. The note states "0700 IV bolus of morphine sulfate 6 mg given as ordered." This is an example of which guideline for recording?
   a. Complete
   b. Organized
   c. Current
   d. Focused

Fill in the blanks in the following questions to reflect the correct legal guidelines for recording.

7. Do not leave a _____ _____ in a narrative note because another person could add incorrect information there.

8. All entries in a chart should be _____ to prevent misinterpretation of information.

9. Correct any _____ promptly to avoid a negative outcome for the patient.

10. When an error has been made in recording, correct it by drawing a _____ through the error.

11. Always chart only for _____ to ensure accountability for information in the record.

12. For each standard time listed below, write the corresponding military time.

    6:23 a.m.

    7:10 p.m.

    12:05 a.m.

    11:55 p.m.

Safe Medication Administration in Practice

Reading Assignment: Administering Medications (Chapter 16)

Patients: Piya Jordan, Medical-Surgical Floor, Room 403
Kathryn Doyle, Skilled Nursing Floor, Room 503

Objectives:

- Discuss the rationale for medications ordered for patients in case studies.
- Explain how to apply the six rights of medication administration.
- Perform medication dosage calculations.
- Explain nursing implications for administering medications.
- Describe potential sources of medication errors.
- Identify factors that influence the selection of form and route of a medication for administration.
- Discuss factors in the case studies that would contraindicate administration of a medication.
- Correctly describe steps for administering a medication.

Overview:

Medication administration is one of the more important responsibilities of a professional nurse because of the risks involved. Any given medication has the potential for creating harmful effects if administered inappropriately or incorrectly. The busy health care environment poses many barriers to safe medication administration. Thus it is important to learn how to attend to the preparation and administration of medications. You can never be too cautious in administering medications. Always follow the six rights of drug administration and be aware of the principles used to calculate and prepare medications safely and accurately. Know the effects that medications may have on your patient's behavior and physical condition so that you can properly monitor the patient and evaluate whether the drugs have been effective.

Patient education is an important part of drug therapy. Patients must obtain the necessary information to self-administer medications safely and know how to monitor their response to medications. Home environments and daily routines influence how patients take their medications. It is important to problem-solve with patients and families to anticipate possible barriers to safe medication administration in the home and workplace.

Exercise 1

  CD-ROM Activity

 45 minutes

In this exercise you will visit Piya Jordan, a 68-year-old Asian-American female who entered the hospital after an emergency department admission for abdominal pain, nausea, and vomiting. She underwent abdominal surgery for the removal of a mass in her right lower quadrant. You may have worked with Piya Jordan previously if you already completed Lesson 10, 12, 14, or 15.

- Sign in to work at Pacific View Regional Hospital on the Medical-Surgical Floor for Period of Care 1. (*Note:* If you are already in the virtual hospital from a previous exercise, click on **Leave the Floor** and then **Restart the Program** to get to the sign-in window.)
- From the Patient List, select Piya Jordan (Room 403).
- Click on **Get Report**.
- Click on **Go to Nurses' Station**.
- Click on **Chart** and then on **403**.
- Click on **History and Physical** and review the information provided.
- Click on **Physician's Orders** and review the orders for Tuesday and Wednesday morning.

1. Piya Jordan has orders for a number of medications postoperatively. Match each medication listed below with the rationale for its administration.

Medication	Rationale
_____ Digoxin 0.125 mg IV	a. Reduce fever
_____ Famotidine 20 mg IV	b. Reduce gastric acid secretion
_____ Cefotetan 1 g IV	c. Slow the heart rate in atrial fibrillation
_____ Acetaminophen 650 mg per rectum q6h	d. Prevent postoperative wound infection

2. Review the physician's postoperative medication orders once again. Are there any dangerous abbreviations used? If so, what is the preferred alternative?

- Once again, review the physician's medication orders for Piya Jordan.
- Now click on **Return to Nurses' Station**.
- Click on the **Medication Room**.
- Select the **MAR** and click on tab **403**.
- Review the MAR for drugs due to be given Wednesday between 0730 and 0815.

3. On the following list, which statements describe activities for correctly following the six rights of medication administration? Select all that apply.

_____ Compare MAR with physician's written order for the name of a medication.

_____ Review the patient record for the patient's allergies.

_____ Review the supply cart for the size of syringes.

_____ Check the MAR against the physician's written order for the route to use to give a medication.

_____ Compare the physician's written order for a medication with the times selected on the MAR for scheduled administration.

→ • Click on **Return to Medication Room**.
  • Based on your care for Piya Jordan, access the various storage areas of the Medication Room to obtain the necessary medications you need to administer.
  • For each area you access, select the medication you plan to administer and then click **Put Medication on Tray**. When finished with a storage area, click on **Close Drawer** or **Close Bin**.
  • Click **View Medication Room**.
  • Click on **Preparation** and choose the correct medication to administer. Click **Prepare**.
  • Follow the Preparation Wizard prompts to prepare the medication. Click **Next** and choose the correct patient to administer this medication to. Click **Finish**.
  • Click on **Review Your Medications** and then on **Return to Medication Room** when ready.

4. How much of the digoxin did you prepare in a syringe for Piya Jordan?

5. Which of the following medications did you prepare for this time period? Select all that apply.

_____ Enoxaparin 40 mg

_____ KCl 20 mEq in 250 mL NS

_____ Digoxin 0.125 mg

_____ Morphine sulfate 2.5 mg per 1 mL

_____ Cefotetan 1 g

• Click on **Nurses' Station**.
- Click on **403** at the bottom of the screen to go to the patient's room.

6. Before you administer digoxin to Piya Jordan, what should you assess?
   a. Blood pressure and IV infusion
   b. Apical heart rate and IV infusion
   c. Potassium level and blood pressure
   d. Patient's level of discomfort and range of motion in knees

7. Before administering the digoxin, what is the main function of the IV infusion you should assess?

 • Perform any necessary assessments and assess any pertinent information before administering your medications.
- After you have collected the appropriate assessment data and are ready for administration, click on **Patient Care** and **Medication Administration**. Verify that the correct patient and medication(s) appear in the left-hand window. Then click the down arrow next to Select. From the drop-down menu, select **Administer** and complete the Administration Wizard by providing any information requested. When the Wizard stops asking for information, click on **Administer to Patient**. Specify **Yes** when asked whether this administration should be recorded in the MAR. Finally, click **Finish**.

8. Indicate whether each of the following statements is true or false.

   a. _____ IV administration of digoxin creates a greater risk to the patient than does IV administration of KCl.

   b. _____ After choosing to hold cefotetan because of Piya Jordan's allergy, you should contact the prescriber immediately.

   c. _____ When you are administering a medication by an intermittent infusion, you should turn off the main IV infusion as the medication is infused.

   d. _____ After administering an intermittent infusion, you should discard the bag of medication and the IV tubing.

9. Why is Piya Jordan not given her digoxin by mouth?

Exercise 2

 CD-ROM Activity

 45 minutes

 In this exercise you will visit Piya Jordan, a 68-year-old Asian-American female who entered the hospital after an emergency department admission for abdominal pain, nausea, and vomiting. She underwent abdominal surgery for the removal of a mass in her right lower quadrant. You may have worked with Piya Jordan previously if you already completed Exercise 1 of this lesson or Lesson 10, 12, 14, or 15.

- Sign in to work at Pacific View Regional Hospital on the Medical-Surgical Floor for Period of Care 2. (*Note:* If you are already in the virtual hospital from a previous exercise, click on **Leave the Floor** and then **Restart the Program** to get to the sign-in window.)
- From the Patient List, select Piya Jordan (Room 403).
- Click on **Get Report**.
- Click on **Go to Nurses' Station**.
- Click on **Chart** and then on **403**.
- Click on **History and Physical** and review.
- Click on **Nurse's Notes** and review.
- Click on and review the **Physician's Orders**.

1. The physician ordered ondansetron 4 mg IV q6h PRN for nausea. Which of the following statements are true about a PRN order?

    _____ It calls for a single dose of a medication to be given only once.

    _____ It is a type of order that requires the medication to be given at a specific time.

    _____ It is an order prescribed for a time when a patient requires it.

    _____ It is the only type of order canceled when a patient goes to surgery.

The physician also ordered enoxaparin 40 mg subQ. Fill in the blanks in the following statements to describe correct principles for administering subcutaneous injections.

2. A subcutaneous injection requires a _____-gauge needle.

3. A _____ to _____-mL syringe is usually adequate for a subcutaneous injection.

4. The best site for administering heparin is the _____.

5. Injecting heparin slowly over 30 seconds may create less _____.

6. Considering Piya Jordan's physical build, what needle length and angle of insertion would you use for the enoxaparin injection?

• Click on **Return to Nurses' Station**.
- Click on **403** at the bottom of the screen.
- Review the **Initial Observations**.
- Click on **Patient Care** and then on **Nurse-Client Interactions**.
- Select and view the video titled **1115: Interventions—Nausea, Blood**. (*Note:* Check the virtual clock to see whether enough time has elapsed. You can use the fast-forward feature to advance the time by 2-minute intervals if the video is not yet available. Then click again on **Patient Care** and **Nurse-Client Interactions** to refresh the screen.)
- Next, click on **Take Vital Signs** at the top of the screen.

7. Based on your review of the physician's medication orders and the nurse-client interaction, do you think it is appropriate to administer the ordered acetaminophen for Piya Jordan? Explain.

8. Piya Jordan has complained of nausea. Go to the Medication Room to prepare ondansetron and then answer the following questions.

   a. The ondansetron comes in a vial/ampule containing how many mL?

   b. What is the correct volume of ondansetron to administer?

 • Click on **Patient Care**.
- Click on **Physical Assessment**.

9. What body system would you assess prior to administering the ondansetron? Explain your answer.

 • Click on **Medication Room** at the bottom of the screen.
- Click on **MAR** and then on tab **403** to determine the medications that Piya Jordan is ordered to receive. (*Note:* While working in the Medication Room, you may click on **Review MAR** at the bottom of the screen at any time to verify the correct medication order. Remember to look at the patient name on the MAR to make sure you have the correct record—you must click on the correct room number within the MAR.)
- Click on **Return to Medication Room** after reviewing the correct MAR.

- Based on your care for Piya Jordan, access the various storage areas of the Medication Room to obtain the necessary medications you need to administer.

- For each area you access, select the medication you plan to administer and then click on **Put Medication on Tray**. When finished with a storage area, click on **Close Drawer** or **Close Bin**.

- Click on **View Medication Room**.

- Click on **Preparation** and choose the correct medication to administer. Click on **Prepare**.

- Click **Next** and choose the correct patient to administer this medication to. Click **Finish**.

- Click on **Review Your Medications** at the bottom of the screen and then on **Return to Medication Room** when ready. Once you are back in the Medication Room, go directly to Piya Jordan's room to administer this medication by clicking on **403** at the bottom of the screen.

- After you have collected the appropriate assessment data and are ready for administration, click on **Patient Care** and on **Medication Administration**. Verify that the correct patient and medication(s) appear in the left-hand window. Then click the down arrow next to Select. From the drop-down menu, select **Administer** and complete the Administration Wizard by providing any information requested. When the Wizard stops asking for information, select **Administer to Patient**. Specify **Yes** when asked whether this administration should be recorded in the MAR. Finally, click **Finish**.

10. Below is a list of steps describing the proper technique for administering an IV push medication. Number the steps from 1 to 10 to indicate the correct sequence in which they should be done.

    _____ Clean injection port with antiseptic swab.

    _____ Recheck fluid infusion rate.

    _____ Perform hand hygiene and apply gloves.

    _____ Select injection port of IV tubing closest to patient.

    _____ Check patient's identification by looking at identification bracelet and asking patient's name.

    _____ Occlude IV line and check for blood return.

    _____ Withdraw syringe from port.

    _____ Connect syringe to IV line.

    _____ Dispose of uncapped needles and syringe and perform hand hygiene.

    _____ Release tubing and inject medication within time recommended.

11. After administering ondansetron, how would you evaluate Piya Jordan for side effects or adverse reactions to the drug?

12. Headache, chest pain, and difficulty breathing can be side effects of ondansetron. If Piya Jordan developed these, what would you do?

13. Checking a patient's identification bracelet before administering a medication ensures that you:
    a. administer the medication at the right time.
    b. administer the medication to the right patient.
    c. administer the right medication.
    d. administer the medication with the right documentation.

Exercise 3

 CD-ROM Activity

 30 minutes

 In this exercise you will visit Kathryn Doyle, a 79-year-old Caucasian female who entered the skilled nursing unit after repair of an intertrochanteric fracture 2 weeks ago. You may have worked with Kathryn Doyle previously if you already completed Lesson 4, 6, or 8.

• Sign in to work at Pacific View Regional Hospital on the Skilled Nursing Floor for Period of Care 2. (*Note:* If you are already in the virtual hospital from a previous exercise, click on **Leave the Floor** and then **Restart the Program** to get to the sign-in window.)
• From the Patient List, select Kathryn Doyle (Room 503).
• Click on **Get Report**.
• Click on **Go to Nurses' Station**.
• Click on **Chart** and then on **503**.
• Click on and review the **History and Physical**.
• Click on and review the **Physician's Orders**.
• Next, click on and review the **Nurse's Notes**.

1. From what you know about Kathryn Doyle from the clinical report, in what way can the administration of oral medications become a useful therapy for one of her clinical problems?

2. Match each of the medications ordered for Kathryn Doyle with its corresponding purpose.

Medication	Purpose
_____ Calcium citrate	a. Treatment for anemia
_____ Ferrous sulfate	b. Prevention of infection
_____ Docusate sodium	c. Prevention of constipation
_____ Ibuprofen	d. Treatment for osteoporosis
	e. Improvement of appetite
	f. Relief of pain in left hip

 • Click on **Return to Nurses' Station**.
  • Click on **Medication Room** at the bottom of the screen.

3. What should you check before beginning to remove medications from the dispensing system? Select all that apply.

_____ Patient's fluid intake for last 8 hours

_____ Patient's vital signs at 0700

_____ Patient's medication administration record

_____ Patient's activity order

_____ Patient's allergy record

• Click on **MAR** and then on tab **503**. Review the patient's MAR to determine the medications that Kathryn Doyle is ordered to receive. (*Note:* When working in the Medication Room, you may click on **Review MAR** at the bottom of the screen at any time to verify the correct medication order. Remember to look at the patient name on the MAR to make sure you have the correct record—you must click on the correct room number within the MAR.)
• Click on **Return to Medication Room** after reviewing the correct MAR.
• Based on your care for Kathryn Doyle, access the various storage areas of the Medication Room to obtain the necessary medications you need to administer.
• For each area you access, select the medication you plan to administer and then click on **Put Medication on Tray**. When finished with a storage area, click on **Close Drawer** or **Close Bin**.
• Click on **View Medication Room**.
• Click on **Preparation** and choose the correct medication to administer. Click **Prepare**.
• Click **Next** and choose the correct patient to administer this medication to. Click **Finish**.
• Click on **Review Your Medications** at the bottom of the screen and then on **Return to Medication Room** when ready.
• Complete questions 4 through 6 below before going to Kathryn Doyle's room to administer her medication.

4. Two of the drugs you are administering to Kathryn Doyle could cause constipation. Which drugs are they?
   a. Ferrous sulfate and docusate sodium
   b. Calcium citrate and ibuprofen
   c. Ibuprofen and ferrous sulfate
   d. Ferrous sulfate and calcium citrate

5. What is the most common side effect to be concerned with when administering ibuprofen?
   a. Gastrointestinal distress
   b. Headache
   c. Black stool
   d. Urinary frequency

6. How many times should you check the information on the MAR against the label on the medication during preparation?

 • Click on **503** at the bottom of the screen to go to Kathryn Doyle's room.
   • Click on **Patient Care**.
   • Click on **Medication Administration**.

7. If Kathryn Doyle asked you to crush her pills and mix them with applesauce, what would be your response?

 • After you have collected the appropriate assessment data and are ready for administration, click on **Patient Care** and **Medication Administration**. Verify that the correct patient and medication(s) appear in the left-hand window.
   • Then click the down arrow next to Select. From the drop-down menu, select **Administer** and complete the Administration Wizard by providing any information requested.
   • When the Wizard stops asking for information, select **Administer to Patient**. Specify **Yes** when asked whether this administration should be recorded in the MAR.
   • Finally, click **Finish**.
   • Now that you have completed administering the medications, click on **Leave the Floor** at the bottom of your screen. From the Floor Menu, select **Look at Your Preceptor's Evaluation**. Then click on **Medication Scorecard**. How did you do? Review your results.

LESSON **8**

Activity and Mobility

OO **Reading Assignment:** Exercise and Activity (Chapter 26)
Immobility (Chapter 35)

Patients: Kathryn Doyle, Skilled Nursing Floor, Room 503
Goro Oishi, Skilled Nursing Floor, Room 505

Objectives:

- Describe the effects of immobility on body systems.
- Describe the effects of exercise on body systems.
- Perform an assessment of a patient's risk for developing complications from immobility.
- Develop a plan of care for promoting activity tolerance in a case study patient.
- Explain nursing interventions appropriate for reducing effects of immobility.
- Describe techniques for safely assisting patients with positioning and ambulation.
- Describe principles for use of assistive devices.

Overview:

Patients within health care settings present a wide variety of activity and mobility limitations. As a nurse, you must be able to recognize not only how patients' presenting health problems affect their ability to remain active and mobile but also how these problems pose risks for the function of all body systems. Preventive care is a key aspect of supporting a patients' mobility and activity tolerance. Early assessment is especially important as you learn to look for changes reflecting the effects of immobilization. As a critical thinker you will learn to incorporate nursing interventions to keep patients active and to prevent complications of immobility.

Exercise 1

 CD-ROM Activity

 45 minutes

 In this exercise you will visit Kathryn Doyle, a 79-year-old Caucasian female who was admitted following a fall at home, in which she sustained a left hip fracture. You may have worked with Kathryn Doyle previously if you already completed Lesson 4, 6, or 7.

- Sign in to work at Pacific View Regional Hospital on the Skilled Nursing Floor for Period of Care 2. (*Note:* If you are already in the virtual hospital from a previous exercise, click on **Leave the Floor** and then **Restart the Program** to get to the sign-in window.)
- From the Patient List, select Kathryn Doyle (Room 503).
- Click on **Get Report**.
- Click on **Go to Nurses' Station**.
- Click on **Chart** and then on **503**.
- Click on and review the **Nursing Admission**.
- Click on and review the **Nurse's Notes**.

1. List three bone and muscle changes that could have resulted from the immobilization of Kathryn Doyle's hip during initial treatment.

2. What factor in Kathryn Doyle's history increased her risk for bone fracture?

3. Using the nursing history as a data base, review the factors that are increasing Kathryn Doyle's risks for complications from immobility. Then, for each of the factors listed below, identify the systemic and psychosocial complications for which she is most at risk.

Risk Factor	Systemic/Psychosocial Complications
Decreased skin turgor	
Limited social support	
Concentrated dark urine	
Limited ROM in left lower leg and reluctance to ambulate	

4. Based on the risks noted in question 3, identify two nursing interventions you would use to minimize the effects of each potential complication.

- Click on **Return to Nurses' Station**.
- Click on **EPR** and then on **Login**.
- Select **503** from the Patient drop-down menu.
- Select **Nutrition** from the Category drop-down menu and review the nutrition findings and then the **Input and Output** data.

Kathryn Doyle's history reveals a poor appetite, and she has not consistently eaten all of her meals. She is at risk for negative nitrogen balance unless she becomes more active and mobile. Use this information to answer questions 5 through 8.

5. In assisting Kathryn Doyle to make dietary selections to avoid a negative nitrogen balance, which of the following will be most beneficial?
   a. Lean meat
   b. Leafy green vegetables
   c. Milk products
   d. Citrus fruits

6. Immobilization causes muscle _____, which leads to negative nitrogen balance.

7. Loss of protein leads to _____ loss.

8. A person who has been immobile and develops a loss of appetite typically has a deficiency

   in calories and _____.

- Click on **Exit EPR**.
- Click on **Chart** and then on **503**.
- Click on **Consultations** and read the Physical Therapy Consult.

9. Why would Kathryn Doyle be given a walker instead of crutches?

10. The physical therapy note states that the left lower extremity is being given ROM. What type of ROM is this likely referring to?

11. While performing ROM exercises on the left lower leg, Kathryn Doyle complains that she is too weak to complete the exercise. What is your best option at this time?
    a. Reduce the number of exercise repetitions.
    b. Have the patient stop exercising and move the joint passively instead.
    c. Stop the exercises until the patient is willing to participate.
    d. Support the leg and foot and coach the patient to move through full ROM as much as she can.

12. When Kathryn Doyle visits physical therapy, the therapists will assist her in walking with a walker and performing ROM exercises. Complete the chart below to describe the evaluation approach for Kathryn Doyle's therapy.

Activity	Evaluation Measures	Expected Responses
Walking with walker		
ROM		

Exercise 2

 CD-ROM Activity

 30 minutes

 In this exercise you will visit Goro Oishi, a 66-year-old Asian-American male who is admitted for hospice care following an intracerebral hemorrhage. You may have worked with Goro Oishi previously if you already completed Lesson 16 or 17.

• Sign in to work at Pacific View Regional Hospital on the Skilled Nursing Floor for Period of Care 1. (*Note:* If you are already in the virtual hospital from a previous exercise, click on **Leave the Floor** and then **Restart the Program** to get to the sign-in window.)
• From the Patient List, select Goro Oishi (Room 505).
• Click on **Get Report**.
• Click on **Go to Nurses' Station**.
• Click on **Chart** and then on **505**.
• Click on and review the **History and Physical**.
• Select **Nursing Admission** and review.

1. Goro Oishi is receiving palliative care, and thus the aim of the nurse is to manage symptoms and minimize the development of discomforting complications. What nursing measure can the nurse initiate that will reduce the patient's risk for pressure ulcer formation and improve his ability to breathe with less effort?

2. Goro Oishi is currently lying on his right side with the head of the bed elevated 20 degrees, and you want to turn him to his left side. Number the steps below from 1 to 13 to indicate the correct sequence in which they should be done. (*Note:* Step 1 has been numbered for you.)

    _____ Place pillow behind patient's back.

    _____ Have each nurse grasp drawsheet firmly near the patient.

    _____ Flex patient's right knee.

    _____ Place pillow under semiflexed right leg level at hip from groin to foot.

    _____ Remove any pillows and roll patient over to assume the supine position.

    __1__ Obtain assistance from another nurse and raise bed to working height.

    _____ Have nurse on left side of bed place one hand on patient's hip and one hand on shoulder; then roll client toward the left.

    _____ Lower side rails and position a nurse on each side of bed.

    _____ Place pillow under patient's head and neck and bring left shoulder blade forward.

    _____ Assuming the proper stance, coordinate with the other nurse and lift the patient to align just to the right side of bed.

    _____ Lower head of bed until it is flat.

    _____ Position both arms in slightly flexed position.

    _____ Place a sandbag parallel to plantar surface of right foot.

3. The clinical report noted that Goro Oishi has an elevated body temperature. Name two ways this can increase the risks associated with immobilization.

Oxygenation

☞ Reading Assignment: Nursing Process (Chapter 8)
                                                Fluid, Electrolyte, and Acid-Base Balances (Chapter 17)
                                                Oxygenation (Chapter 29)

Patients: Patricia Newman, Medical-Surgical Floor, Room 406
                      Jacquline Catanazaro, Medical-Surgical Floor, Room 402

Objectives:

- Describe factors that can alter oxygenation.
- Explain the relationship between cardiac and respiratory alterations.
- Identify the influence that physiologic changes in oxygenation have on a patient's clinical condition.
- Identify lifestyle risk factors for problems with oxygenation.
- Apply critical thinking in the assessment of a case study patient.
- Identify nursing diagnoses that apply to a case study patient.
- Explain the rationale for use of specific nursing interventions for patients in the case studies.
- Identify the proper approach to evaluate a patient's responses to oxygenation therapies.

Overview:

The normal function of the cardiac and respiratory systems in delivering oxygen is necessary to sustain life. In the care of patients with oxygenation alterations, it is important for you as the nurse to understand cardiovascular and respiratory physiology. This knowledge base will allow you to better understand assessment data, select appropriate nursing diagnoses, and plan relevant nursing interventions.

Changes in a patient's oxygenation can be the result of acute or chronic disease conditions. Patients in acute respiratory distress will be anxious and fearful, requiring your timely and attentive care. Patients with chronic respiratory disorders will require your support in understanding the long-term implications of an illness and your assistance in adapting their lifestyle.

Exercise 1

 CD-ROM Activity

 45 minutes

 Patricia Newman is a 61-year-old Caucasian female with a history of emphysema for 12 years. She has been admitted to the emergency department in moderate respiratory distress. You may have worked with Patricia Newman previously if you already completed Lesson 2, 3, 5, or 10.

- Sign in to work at Pacific View Regional Hospital on the Medical-Surgical Floor for Period of Care 1. (*Note:* If you are already in the virtual hospital from a previous exercise, click on **Leave the Floor** and then **Restart the Program** to get to the sign-in window.)
- From the Patient List, select Patricia Newman (Room 406).
- Click on **Get Report** and review the clinical report summary.
- Click on **Go to Nurses' Station**.
- Click on **Chart** and then on **406**.
- Click on and review the **History and Physical**.
- Click on and review the patient's **Laboratory Reports**.

1. Patricia Newman is 61 years old. Let's assume that she has smoked since the age of 22. If so, how many packs of cigarettes would she have averaged on a daily basis? (*Study Tip:* Apply the formula for pack-year history.)

2. Patricia Newman has been diagnosed with pneumonia. Which of the following physiologic changes in oxygenation result from pneumonia? Select all that apply.

_____ Impaired ventilatory movement

_____ Decreased hemoglobin level

_____ Decreased diffusion of oxygen from the alveoli to the blood

_____ Inability of tissues to extract oxygen from the blood

_____ Obstruction of airways with mucus

3. Patricia Newman also has emphysema, a form of chronic obstructive pulmonary disease. Below, provide a rationale for each of the listed physiologic changes that result from emphysema.

Physiologic Change	Rationale
Increased work of breathing	
Fatigue	
Dyspnea on exertion	
Elevated $PaCO_2$	

→ • While still in the patient's chart, review the **Nursing Admission**.

4. As you review the data in Patricia Newman's History and Physical and Nursing Admission, apply the critical thinking model in your assessment of the patient. Complete the following critical thinking diagram for assessment of Patricia Newman's situation by writing the letter of each critical thinking factor under its proper category.

Knowledge

1. _____

2. _____

3. _____

Experience	**ASSESSMENT OXYGENATION**	**Attitudes**
4. _____		6. _____
5. _____		7. _____
	Standards	

8. _____

9. _____

10. _____

Critical Thinking Factors

a. Patricia Newman shows a pattern of poor health promotion practices. Explore and learn more about the patient to understand the reason for her behavior.

b. Apply what you know about respiratory physiology to determine the effects emphysema has on rate and depth of breathing.

c. The time you cared for a patient with pneumonia in the health clinic previously will help you recognize Patricia Newman's presenting symptoms.

d. Compare the ranges of normal laboratory values with Patricia Newman's test results.

e. Each time you auscultate lung sounds, be sure to follow the same pattern for placement of the stethoscope as you listen to all lobes of the lung.

f. Refer to nutrition therapy principles when you assess the patient's diet history.

g. If you are uncertain about how to interpret arterial blood gas levels, read a reference on acid-base balance.

h. Reflect on the time you cared for a patient with emphysema in the past. How did that patient adjust to the need to follow a medication schedule, and what is similar about Patricia Newman?

i. Refer to pharmacology sources in reviewing the effects of Patricia Newman's medications on her blood pressure.

j. When auscultating the patient's blood pressure, be sure the cuff is applied correctly to her arm and that you inflate the cuff 30 mm Hg above point at which palpable pulse disappears.

• Click on **Return to Nurses' Station**.
- Click on **406** at the bottom of the screen.
- Review the **Initial Observations.**
- Click on **Patient Care**.
- Click on **Physical Assessment** and review the assessments for Head & Neck, Chest, and Back & Spine.

5. When auscultating Patricia Newman's lung sounds, what sounds would you expect as a result of pneumonia? Give a rationale.

6. Patricia Newman has sinus tachycardia as a result of which of the following factors? Select all that apply.

_____ Tobacco use

_____ Estrogen patch use

_____ Pain

_____ Hypoxia

_____ Hypertension

7. Patricia Newman's assessment reveals the following physical findings: $PaCO_2$ 47; dyspnea on exertion; naps frequently; abnormal rate and depth of breathing. Based on these findings, what is the most appropriate nursing diagnosis?
   a. Ineffective breathing pattern
   b. Ineffective tissue perfusion
   c. Impaired gas exchange
   d. Ineffective airway clearance

8. Give a rationale for the nursing diagnosis you chose in question 7.

9. For the nursing diagnosis of Impaired Gas Exchange, list two outcomes that you would develop in a plan of care to address the goal of "Patient will experience improved gas exchange."

10. What is the stimulus for Patricia Newman to breathe? What is the normal stimulus to breathe?

Exercise 2

 CD-ROM Activity

 30 minutes

 Patricia Newman is a 61-year-old Caucasian female with a history of emphysema for 12 years. She has been admitted to the emergency department in moderate respiratory distress. You may have worked with Patricia Newman previously if you completed Exercise 1 of this lesson or Lesson 2, 3, 5, or 10.

- Sign in to work at Pacific View Regional Hospital on the Medical-Surgical Floor for Period of Care 2. (*Note:* If you are already in the virtual hospital from a previous exercise, click on **Leave the Floor** and then **Restart the Program** to get to the sign-in window.)
- From the Patient List, select Patricia Newman (Room 406).
- Click on **Get Report** and review.
- Click on **Go to Nurses' Station**.
- Click on **Chart** and then on **406**.
- Review the **History and Physical**.

1. Complete the chart below for Patricia Newman's arterial blood gas values. (*Study Tip:* Review acid-base balance in Chapter 17 in your textbook.)

Blood Gas Value	Normal or Abnormal?	Reason for Abnormal Values
pH 7.33		
PaO$_2$ 70		
HCO$_3$ 26		
CO$_2$ 47		

2. List three lifestyle risk factors that likely contribute to Patricia Newman's emphysema and hypertension.

 • Review the **Nursing Admission**.

3. Patricia Newman's history reveals poor adherence to health promotion behaviors. As her nurse, what recommendations might you make to prevent future occurrences of pneumonia?

• Click on **Return to Nurses' Station**.
• Click on **406** at the bottom of the screen to go to Patricia Newman's room.
• Review the **Initial Observations.**
• Click on **Patient Care** and then on **Nurse-Client Interactions**.
• Select and view the video titled **1100: Care Coordination**. (*Note:* Check the virtual clock to see whether enough time has elapsed. You can use the fast-forward feature to advance the time by 2-minute intervals if the video is not yet available. Then click again on **Patient Care** and **Nurse-Client Interactions** to refresh the screen.)

4. Patricia Newman has a number of health problems. Listed below are nursing diagnoses that apply to her. Draw a concept map in the figure provided by showing the connection between the nursing diagnoses. (*Study Tip:* See pages 132 through 134 in your textbook.)

Impaired Gas Exchange

Fatigue

Imbalanced Nutrition: Less Than Body Requirements

Ineffective Health Maintenance

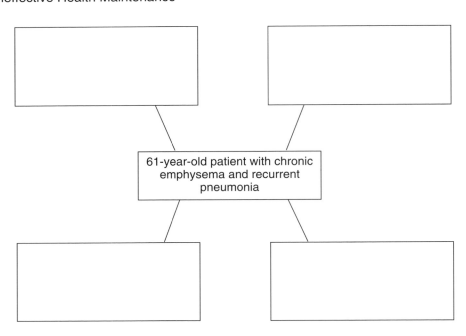

→ • Click on **Chart** and then on **406**.
  • Click on and review the **Patient Education** file.

5. Match each recommended therapy below with its corresponding rationale.

Therapy	Rationale
_____ Use metered-dose inhaler	a. Promotes airway clearance
_____ Perform pursed-lip breathing	b. Reduces degree of dyspnea
_____ Increase periods of walking to 20 minutes 2 times a day	c. Dilates airways, reducing airflow resistance
_____ Perform effective cascade cough	d. Maintains normal mucociliary clearance
_____ Increase fluids to 3 liters per day	e. Prevents alveolar collapse

6. In addition to pursed-lip breathing, what other breathing exercise might you teach Patricia Newman? Explain.

7. Patricia Newman is receiving oxygen 2 liters per minute by nasal cannula. Based on this information, indicate whether each of the following questions is true or false.

a. _____ Increasing the flow rate on a nasal cannula oxygen device to 6 liters per minute will significantly increase delivered oxygen concentration.

b. _____ A flow rate of 2 liters per minute delivers approximately 24% to 28% oxygen.

c. _____ An oxygen mask is a delivery device that would be contraindicated for Patricia Newman.

d. _____ When placing patients on oxygen, you should attach a humidified oxygen source to reduce nasal mucosal drying.

e. _____ Because Patricia Newman's PaO_2 is 70, she might benefit from receiving oxygen by a Venturi mask.

Exercise 3

 CD-ROM Activity

 30 minutes

 Jacquline Catanazaro is a 45-year-old female with a 30-year history of asthma, complicated by schizophrenia. She has been admitted to the ED because of an acute asthma episode and concurrent schizophrenic episode. You may have worked with Jacquline Catanazaro previously if you completed Lesson 13 or 14.

• Sign in to work at Pacific View Regional Hospital on the Medical-Surgical Floor for Period of Care 1. (*Note:* If you are already in the virtual hospital from a previous exercise, click on **Leave the Floor** and then **Restart the Program** to get to the sign-in window.)
• From the Patient List, select Jacquline Catanazaro (Room 402).
• Click on **Get Report**.
• Click on **Go to Nurses' Station**.
• Click on **Chart** and then on **402**.
• Click on and review the **Nursing Admission**.

1. Explain how Jacquline Catanazaro's obesity affects her ability to breathe.

2. Jacquline Catanazaro reportedly can become very anxious from her mental illness. Which of the following best describes the influence anxiety has on the patient's oxygenation status?
   a. Causes hypoventilation
   b. Increases the body's metabolic rate and oxygen demand
   c. Reduces the diffusion of oxygen across the alveolar membrane
   d. Creates a sense of breathlessness from CO_2 retention

3. The physician ordered stat nebulization for Jacquline Catanazaro using albuterol. Nebulization will most likely improve her ability to breathe by what mechanism(s)? Select all that apply. (*Study Tip:* Refer to your pharmacology textbook for albuterol's action.)

   _____ Decreasing the volume of sputum to expectorate

   _____ Cooling inhaled air

   _____ Relieving bronchospasm

   _____ Enhancing mucociliary clearance

   _____ Reducing the patient's peak flow rate

 • Click on **Return to Nurses' Station**.
   • Select **402** at the bottom of the screen.
   • Review the **Initial Observations.**
   • Click on **Patient Care** and then **Nurse-Client Interactions**.
   • Select and view the video titled **0730: Intervention—Airway**. (*Note:* Check the virtual clock to see whether enough time has elapsed. You can use the fast-forward feature to advance the time by 2-minute intervals if the video is not yet available. Then click again on **Patient Care** and **Nurse-Client Interactions** to refresh the screen.)
   • Next, click on **Physical Assessment** and conduct a focused assessment based on Jacquline Catanazaro's current condition.

4. Match Jacquline Catanazaro's physical findings with its corresponding physiologic change.

Physical Finding	**Physiologic Change**
_____ Hyperresonance to percussion	a. Increased airway resistance
_____ Substernal retraction	b. High-velocity airflow
_____ Tachypnea	c. Air-filled lungs
_____ Wheezes bilaterally	d. Decreased oxygen levels trigger increased respiratory rate
_____ Peak flow meter shows value of 200	e. Increased work of breathing

• Click on **Leave the Floor**.
- From the Floor Menu, select **Restart the Program**.
- Sign in to work on the Medical-Surgical Floor for Period of Care 2.
- From the Patient List, select Jacquline Catanazaro (Room 402).
- Click on **Go to Nurses' Station**.
- Click on **Chart** and then on **402**.
- Select the **Physician's Notes** and review.
- Select the **Physician's Orders** and review.

5. The physician's notes for 0800 and 1000 show two sets of arterial blood gas results:

   0800: pH 7.38, PaO_2 80, $PaCO_2$ 50, HCO_3 26, oxygen saturation 85%

   1000: pH 7.40, PaO_2 92, $PaCO_2$ 40, HCO_3 23, oxygen saturation 99%

   a. Explain the reason for the change in this patient's blood gases.

   b. Are Jacquline Catanazaro's ABGs now normal?

6. Considering that Jacquline Catanazaro has a productive cough with frothy secretions, why would it be inadvisable to perform tracheal suctioning?

LESSON **10** _____

Managing Fluid and Electrolyte Balance

_____

Reading Assignment: Fluids, Electrolyte, and Acid-Base Balances (Chapter 17)
Oxygenation (Chapter 29)
Surgical Patient (Chapter 38)

Patients: Piya Jordan, Medical-Surgical Floor, Room 403
Patricia Newman, Medical-Surgical Floor, Room 406

Objectives:

- Identify disturbances in fluids and electrolytes in case study patients.
- Identify acid-base imbalances in case study patients.
- Explain the function of electrolytes.
- Apply critical thinking in the assessment of a patient for fluid and electrolyte imbalance.
- Describe variables that affect fluid and electrolyte balance.
- Describe factors to include in the assessment of a peripheral intravenous site.
- Calculate an intravenous flow rate.
- Describe the risks associated with blood transfusion.
- Identify steps used in the insertion of a peripheral intravenous catheter.

Overview:

Fluid, electrolyte and acid-base balances within the body are needed to maintain the health and function of all body systems. As a nurse it is important to understand what physiologic changes occur from fluid and electrolyte and acid-base imbalances, the risks a patient has for imbalance, and the types of therapies used to reverse imbalance. An important responsibility is to monitor patients closely for fluid and electrolyte or acid-base changes. A patient's condition can change very quickly, thus requiring a nurse's astute observation and timely action.

Competency in the safe and effective administration of intravenous fluid therapy is critical to management of fluid and electrolyte and acid-base alterations. This includes knowing how to correctly establish IV access, monitoring and calculating IV infusions, and maintaining infusion systems. How well you manage IV infusion therapy may determine your patient's clinical course.

127

Exercise 1

  CD-ROM Activity

 45 minutes

In this exercise you will visit Piya Jordan, a 68-year-old Asian-American female who entered the hospital after an emergency department admission for abdominal pain, nausea, and vomiting. She underwent abdominal surgery for the removal of a mass in her right lower quadrant. You may have worked with Piya Jordan previously if you already completed Lesson 7, 12, 14, or 15.

- Sign in to work at Pacific View Regional Hospital on the Medical-Surgical Floor for Period of Care 1. (*Note:* If you are already in the virtual hospital from a previous exercise, click on **Leave the Floor** and then **Restart the Program** to get to the sign-in window.)
- From the Patient List, select Piya Jordan (Room 403).
- Click on **Get Report**.
- Click on **Go to Nurses' Station**.
- Click on **Chart** and then on **403**.
- Review the **Nursing Admission**.

1. Identify three factors in Piya Jordan's Nursing Admission data that explain her risks for fluid and electrolyte imbalance prior to surgery.

2. Consider the data you received from the clinical report summary. From the following list, identify the risks Piya Jordan has for fluid and electrolyte imbalance postoperatively. Select all that apply.

_____ Taking digoxin at home

_____ Nasogastric tube draining moderate brown fluid

_____ Intravenous infusion of D_5NS with 20 mEq KCl

_____ Receiving meperidine via patient-controlled analgesia

_____ Being NPO

_____ Telemetry shows atrial fibrillation

• Still in the chart, click on **Laboratory Reports** and review the chemistry findings.

3. Complete the chart below by listing Piya Jordan's chemistry results. Note whether values show a normal or abnormal trend.

Lab Value	Mon 2200	Tues 0630	Wed 0630	Normal/Abnormal?
Na				
K				
Cl				
CO_2				
BUN				

4. As a result of Piya Jordan's trend toward hypokalemia, which of the following signs and symptoms would she most likely experience? Select all that apply.

_____ Confusion

_____ Abnormal ventricular arrhythmias

_____ Flushed skin

_____ Weakness and fatigue

_____ Thirst

_____ Decreased bowel sounds

_____ Diarrhea

• Click on and review the **History and Physical**.

5. Piya Jordan's BUN is elevated. The BUN is a measure of urea in the blood and is an indication of the excretory function of the kidney. Why might the BUN be elevated preoperatively? What treatment did she receive to help reverse this?

6. Piya Jordan's postoperative care will require you as the nurse to conduct a thorough assessment. Critical thinking applied to assessment enables a nurse to develop a relevant plan of care. Complete the following critical thinking diagram for assessment of Piya Jordan's situation by writing the letter of each critical thinking factor under its proper category.

Knowledge

1. _____

2. _____

3. _____

Experience   **PLANNING**   **Standards**

4. _____

5. _____

6. _____

7. _____

Attitudes

8. _____

Critical Thinking Factors

a. Be very thorough in your approach to assessment, take time to examine the abdominal wound and dressing, and do not rush yourself.
b. When measuring Piya Jordan's output from the JP tube, use a measured container.
c. Review the physiology of the effect that surgery has on fluid and electrolyte balance.
d. Consider how a surgical alteration of the colon will affect fluid and electrolyte balance.
e. As you assess Piya Jordan, consider the appearance of the skin and mucous membranes in previous patients you have cared for.
f. Refer to the Infusion Nurse's Society infiltration and phlebitis scales when examining Piya Jordan's IV site.
g. Be aware of normal physical assessment findings as you compare findings from your examination of Piya Jordan.
h. Consider what you know about signs and symptoms of electrolyte alterations.

→ • Click on **Return to Nurses' Station**.
• Click on **403** at the bottom of the screen.
• Review the **Initial Observations.**

7. Piya Jordan's IV is running at 100 mL/hr. Assuming the IV is being delivered via a macro-drip tube, compute the drop rates for each of the two different drop factors below.

Drop factor	Drop rate (gtt/mL)
IV drop factor 10 gtt/mL	
IV drop factor 15 gtt/mL	

8. Piya Jordan's physician has ordered D5 1/2 NS to run at 100 mL/hr. This fluid can best be described as:
   a. isotonic.
   b. hypotonic.
   c. normotonic.
   d. hypertonic.

 • Click on **Patient Care**.

• Click on **Physical Assessment**.

• Review the assessment categories that you believe pertain to Piya Jordan's fluid and electrolyte status.

9. During Piya Jordan's Head & Neck assessment, the subcategories of Gastrointestinal and Integumentary reveal the following: oral mucosa pink and moist, skin warm and moist. What do these findings indicate?

10. Observe the photo of Piya Jordan's IV site during the Upper Extremities assessment. What is wrong with the dressing?

11. Which of the following best describes an IV site without complications?
    a. IV infusing at 75 mL/hr, site warm with redness, nontender
    b. IV infusing at 100 mL/hr, site nontender, without redness or swelling
    c. IV infusing at keep-vein-open rate, swelling less than 1 inch around site, cool to touch
    d. IV infusing at 100 mL/hr, pain on palpation over site, skin blanched and cool to touch

 • Click on the **EPR** and then **Login**.

• Select **403** from the Patient drop-down menu and **Intake and Output** from the Category drop-down menu.

• Review the Intake and Output for Piya Jordan between 2300 on Tuesday and 0700 Wednesday.

12. What was Piya Jordan's fluid balance (intake minus output) for the 8-hour period 2300 to 0700?

13. Which of the following interventions would be appropriate in Piya Jordan's case to manage the fluid imbalance?
    a. Give the patient oral liquids
    b. Increase the infusion rate of the IV
    c. Give the patient tube feeding
    d. Discontinue NG decompression

Exercise 2

 CD-ROM Activity

 45 minutes

 In this exercise you will visit Piya Jordan, a 68-year-old Asian-American female who entered the hospital after an emergency department admission for abdominal pain, nausea, and vomiting. She underwent abdominal surgery for the removal of a mass in her right lower quadrant. You may have worked with Piya Jordan previously if you already completed Exercise 1 of this lesson or Lesson 7, 12, 14, or 15.

- Sign in to work at Pacific View Regional Hospital on the Medical-Surgical Floor for Period of Care 2. (*Note:* If you are already in the virtual hospital from a previous exercise, click on **Leave the Floor** and then **Restart the Program** to get to the sign-in window.)
- From the Patient List, select Piya Jordan (Room 403).
- Click on **Get Report**.
- Click on **Go to Nurses' Station**.
- Click on **Chart** and then on **403**.
- Click on **History and Physical** and review.
- Next, click on **Physician's Orders** and review.
- Finally, click on **Laboratory Reports** and review.

1. The surgeon has ordered 2 units of packed red blood cells to be administered to Piya Jordan for a low hemoglobin and hematocrit. What caused the drop in her hemoglobin and hematocrit?

2. The laboratory reports indicate that Piya Jordan's blood type is A+. Complete the chart below by filling in each box as it applies to Piya Jordan.

Patient's Blood Type	Red Blood Cell Antigen	Transfuse with Type A?	Transfuse with Type B?	Transfuse with Type AB?	Transfuse with Type O?

3. What does the positive symbol (+) indicate for Piya Jordan's blood type?

• Still in the chart, click on the **Nurse's Notes**.

4. The nurse's notes indicate that the nurse "explained precautions" related to blood procurement. Which of the following is the correct procedure to ensure a patient receives the right blood product?
   a. When checking the blood label, have the nurse administering the blood check the patient's name.
   b. When checking the blood label, have two designated staff check the label for the blood type.
   c. When checking the blood label, have two designated staff check it against the patient's name, identification number, and the blood type.
   d. When checking the label, have the nurse administering the blood ask the patient to identify his or her blood type.

5. The physician orders a saline lock to be inserted for the administration of 2 units of packed cells. Number the steps below from 1 to 13 to show the correct sequence for inserting a saline lock.

   _____ Release tourniquet temporarily.

   _____ Look for blood return and advance catheter into vein; loosen and remove stylet.

   _____ Prepare an IV bag, tubing, and saline lock, filling tubing and lock with normal saline.

   _____ Select a vein large enough for catheter placement. Palpate vein and promote venous distention.

   _____ Perform hand hygiene.

   _____ Perform venipuncture. Puncture skin and vein, holding catheter at 10- to 30-degree angle. Insert with bevel up.

   _____ Stabilize the catheter, apply pressure above insertion site, and release tourniquet.

   _____ Apply disposable gloves.

   _____ Reapply tourniquet.

   _____ Identify an accessible vein; apply tourniquet.

   _____ Cleanse insertion site.

   _____ Connect adapter from fluid infusion tubing and saline lock to catheter hub.

   _____ Release roller clamp and regulate infusion rate.

6. Before a transfusion begins, the nurse obtains a patient's baseline _____ signs.

7. The initiation of a transfusion begins _____ to allow for early detection of a transfusion reaction.

8. The nurse stays with a patient during the first _____ minutes, the time when a transfusion reaction is most likely to occur.

9. A unit of packed RBCs should be transfused over a period of _____ hours.

10. If the patient develops chills, fever, tachycardia, or tachypnea, the first action is to

    _____ the transfusion.

Exercise 3

CD-ROM Activity

30 minutes

Patricia Newman is a 61-year-old Caucasian female with a history of emphysema for 12 years. She has been admitted to the emergency department in moderate respiratory distress. You may have worked with Patricia Newman previously if you already completed Lesson 2, 3, 5, or 9.

- Sign in to work at Pacific View Regional Hospital on the Medical-Surgical Floor for Period of Care 1. (*Note:* If you are already in the virtual hospital from a previous exercise, click on **Leave the Floor** and then **Restart the Program** to get to the sign-in window.)
- From the Patient List, select Patricia Newman (Room 406).
- Click on **Get Report**.
- Click on **Go to Nurses' Station**.
- Click on **Chart** and then on **406**.
- Review the **Nursing Admission**.

1. The clinical report summary reveals the following blood gas findings: pH 7.33, O_2 70, HCO_3 26, CO_2 47, O_2 sat 92%

   a. Answer the questions below to help you determine what type of acid-base imbalance this indicates.

   pH = _____

   Acidosis or alkalosis? _____

   Patient's primary physical alteration is metabolic or respiratory? _____

   If source of imbalance is metabolic, expect:

If source of imbalance is respiratory, expect:

b. The type of imbalance is:

 • Click on the **History and Physical**.

2. What condition has originally caused Patricia Newman to have this alteration in blood gases?
   a. Hypertension
   b. Emphysema
   c. Low flow of oxygen via cannula
   d. Pneumonia

3. Alteration in respiratory function can be caused by three different primary alterations. Which of these apply to the emphysema affecting Patricia Newman?
   a. Hypoventilation
   b. Hyperventilation
   c. Hypoxia

4. Patricia Newman's pneumonia complicates her respiratory condition by causing which of the following?
   a. Hypoventilation
   b. Hyperventilation
   c. Hypoxia

5. What physiologic stimulus causes Patricia Newman to breathe? (*Study Tip:* Review pages 802 through 803 in your textbook.)

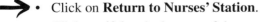 • Click on **Return to Nurses' Station**.
   • Click on **406** at the bottom of the screen to go to Patricia Newman's room.
   • Review the **Initial Observations.**
   • Click on **Patient Care**.
   • Select and review the physical assessments of the **Chest & Back** and the **Spine**.

6. Which of the following symptoms is most likely to be the result of respiratory acidosis?
   a. Mild dyspnea
   b. Normal heart sounds
   c. Sinus tachycardia
   d. Coarse crackles

→ • Click on **Chart** and then on **406**.
   • Review the **Physician's Orders**.
   • Review the **Patient Education** notes.

7. To better manage the patient's acid-base imbalance, the nurse will attempt to improve Patricia Newman's oxygenation. Match each nursing interventions below with its corresponding rationale.

Nursing Intervention	Rationale
_____ Encourage effective coughing	a. Opens bronchioles to enhance oxygen and carbon dioxide exchange
_____ Instruct patient to perform pursed-lip breathing	b. Relieves hypoxia and helps to minimize dyspnea
_____ Administer bronchodilator by metered-dose inhaler	c. Removes secretions that alter diffusion of O_2 and CO_2
_____ Promote fluid intake	d. Reduces thick tenacious secretions that hinder gas diffusion
_____ Administer O_2 at 2 liters per nasal cannula	e. Prevents alveolar collapse and thus improves O_2 diffusion

LESSON 11

Sleep

○Ͽ **Reading Assignment:** Oxygenation (Chapter 29)
Sleep (Chapter 30)
Nutrition (Chapter 32)

Patients: Pablo Rodriguez, Medical-Surgical Floor, Room 405
William Jefferson, Skilled Nursing Floor, Room 501

Objectives:

- Identify factors that disrupt sleep in case study patients.
- Describe the relationship between disturbed sleep pattern and other nursing diagnoses.
- Develop a plan of care to promote sleep for a case study patient.
- Describe interventions designed to promote sleep.
- Identify approaches used to evaluate a patient's sleep status.

Overview:

Proper rest and sleep are essential to good health. As a nurse you will care for patients who often have preexisting sleep disturbances or who develop sleep problems as a result of illness or the experience of hospitalization. To best assist patients, you must understand the nature of sleep, the factors influencing it, and a client's sleep habits. Each patient is unique in regard to his or her sleep pattern. Patients require an individualized approach based on personal habits and pattern of sleep, as well as the particular problems influencing sleep. Your intervention can be effective in resolving both short-term and long-term sleep problems.

137

Exercise 1

  CD-ROM Activity

 45 minutes

In this exercise you will visit Pablo Rodriguez, a 71-year-old Hispanic male who is suffering from advanced non-small cell lung carcinoma. You may have worked with Pablo Rodriguez previously if you already completed Lesson 6, 12, 13, or 19.

* Sign in to work at Pacific View Regional Hospital on the Medical-Surgical Floor for Period of Care 1. (*Note:* If you are already in the virtual hospital from a previous exercise, click on **Leave the Floor** and then **Restart the Program** to get to the sign-in window.)
* From the Patient List, select Pablo Rodriguez (Room 405).
* Click on **Get Report**.
* Click on **Go to Nurses' Station**.
* Click on **Chart** and then on **405**.
* Click on the **Nursing Admission** and review.

1. From the list below, identify the factors in Pablo Rodriguez's history that are contributing to his sleep problem. Select all that apply.

   _____ Eats spicy cheese and refried beans

   _____ Smoked 60 pack years

   _____ Depression

   _____ Takes celecoxib at home

   _____ Pain from subcutaneous nodules

   _____ Dyspnea when lying flat

2. Pablo Rodriguez reports "poor sleep and restlessness" when admitted to the hospital. His Nursing Admission notes that he sleeps 6 to 8 hours and then naps 1 to 2 times a day. List three questions to ask to better clarify his sleep pattern.

 * Click on **Return to Nurses' Station**.
* Click on Room **405** at the bottom of the screen.
* Click on **Patient Care** and then **Nurse-Client Interactions**.
* Select and view the video titled **0730: Symptom Management**. (*Note:* Check the virtual clock to see whether enough time has elapsed. You can use the fast-forward feature to advance the time by 2-minute intervals if the video is not yet available. Then click again on **Patient Care** and **Nurse-Client Interactions** to refresh the screen.)

3. Pablo Rodriguez is obviously experiencing emotional distress as a result of his illness. Information from his Nursing Admission further confirms this. With this information in mind, indicate whether each of the following statements is true or false.

a. _____ Emotional stress may cause a person to try too hard to fall asleep.

b. _____ Older adults who experience depressive moods often have later appearance of REM sleep.

c. _____ Depression can cause a person to have frequent and early awakening.

4. Listed below are signs and symptoms revealed in Pablo Rodriguez's Nursing Admission and initial clinical summary. Group the signs and symptoms into four clusters reflecting four different health problems. To form the clusters, number each of the signs or symptoms with a 1, 2, 3, or 4 to indicate which group it belongs to.

Signs and Symptoms

_____ Labored breathing

_____ Verbal complaint of not feeling rested

_____ Aversion to food from smell of food

_____ Pain reported as 8 on scale of 0 to 10

_____ Trouble falling asleep

_____ Nausea

_____ Dyspnea when lying flat

_____ Nodules painful to palpation

_____ Awakens after falling asleep

_____ Facial mask with expression of discomfort

_____ Tachypneic

5. Now that you have clustered the signs and symptoms (or defining characteristics), which of the following nursing diagnoses are most appropriate for Pablo Rodriguez?
   a. Fatigue; Pain; Imbalanced Nutrition: Less Than Body Requirements; Sleep Disturbance
   b. Pain; Sleep Disturbance; Anxiety; Nausea
   c. Impaired Gas Exchange; Fatigue; Nausea; Anxiety
   d. Impaired Gas Exchange; Pain; Nausea; Sleep Disturbance

6. Given Pablo Rodriguez's numerous physical problems, develop a concept map by drawing arrows to show the association between nursing diagnoses.

 • Click on **Patient Care** and then **Nurse-Client Interactions**.
   • While you are still in Pablo Rodriguez's room, select and view the video titled **0735: Patient Perceptions**. (*Note:* Check the virtual clock to see whether enough time has elapsed. You can use the fast-forward feature to advance the time by 2-minute intervals if the video is not yet available. Then click again on **Patient Care** and **Nurse-Client Interactions** to refresh the screen.)

7. For the nursing diagnosis of Disturbed Sleep Pattern, identify four possible related factors.

8. Pablo Rodriguez's sleep problem is best described as:
   a. sleep apnea.
   b. insomnia.
   c. sleep deprivation.
   d. excessive daytime sleepiness.

9. Develop a nursing plan of care for this nursing diagnosis: Disturbed Sleep Pattern related to pain, nausea, depression, and dyspnea. In the care plan below, fill in additional goals, outcomes, interventions, and rationales. (*Study Tip:* Review Chapters 29 and 32 in your textbook for interventions and rationales.)

Nursing Diagnosis:
Disturbed Sleep Pattern related to pain, nausea, depression, and dyspnea

Goals	Outcomes
1. Patient will achieve an improved sense of sleep	1.
2.	2. Patient will report being able to sleep 6 hours in hospital
	3.

Interventions	Rationales
1. Keep HOB elevated, turn patient in position of comfort and	1.
2.	2. Relief of pain and nausea eliminate physiologic distractions that cause wakefulness
3.	3. Relieves nausea
4. Use culturally appropriate approach in helping patient to discuss concerns over family upon his death	4.

---

10. After instituting your plan of care, what three evaluation measures could you use to determine whether Pablo Rodriguez's sleep disturbance has been resolved?

Exercise 2

 CD-ROM Activity

 45 minutes

 In this exercise you will visit William Jefferson, a 75-year-old African-American male who has a history of Alzheimer's disease and various other chronic ailments. He has been admitted to the skilled nursing unit with a urinary tract infection and possible sepsis. You may have worked with William Jefferson previously if you already completed Lesson 19.

- Sign in to work at Pacific View Regional Hospital on the Skilled Nursing Floor for Period of Care 1. (*Note:* If you are already in the virtual hospital from a previous exercise, click on **Leave the Floor** and then **Restart the Program** to get to the sign-in window.)
- From the Patient List, select William Jefferson (Room 501).
- Click on **Get Report**.
- Click on **Go to Nurses' Station**.
- Click on **Chart** and then on **501**.
- Click on **Nursing Admission** and review.

1. William Jefferson is reported by his wife to have some difficulty with sleeping at home. What food preferences, if eaten in the evening, might be altering his ability to fall asleep?

2. Mrs. Jefferson reports that she does not let her husband nap for more than 1 hour. What would be your response to this information?

→ - Click on and review the **Physician's Orders**.

3. Which of the following medications may contribute to William Jefferson's sleep problem. Select all that apply. (*Study Tip:* Refer to your pharmacology text for a complete list of medications that affect sleep.)

_____ Rivastigmine tartrate

_____ Ibuprofen

_____ Hydrochlorothiazide

_____ Enalapril maleate

_____ Ciprofloxacin

_____ Metformin

_____ Atenolol

4. Explain the rationale for hydrochlorothiazide affecting a patient's sleep. Does William Jefferson's history confirm such a problem?

5. Knowing the effects of the medications on William Jefferson's sleep, what action might you take?

6. Indicate whether each of the following statements is true or false.

   a. _____   Low noises within the extended-care facility, such as staff talking outside of a room, are more likely to arouse a person from stage 3 sleep.

   b. _____   A room that is too hot can cause a person to be restless and unable to fall asleep.

   c. _____   It may take up to 2 weeks before elimination of a food from the diet can restore sleep.

   d. _____   The herbal product Kava can cause insomnia.

7. Match each sleep intervention with its corresponding rationale.

Intervention	**Rationale**
_____ Have Mrs. Jefferson offer chamomile tea to her husband in the evening.	a. Promotes maximal ventilation
_____ Recommend that William Jefferson wear loose-fitting nightwear to bed.	b. Maintains a state of fatigue and promotes relaxation
_____ Recommend a low-running fan in the bedroom at night.	c. Prevents discomfort of full bladder
_____ Encourage the patient and his wife to take their dog for a walk 2 hours before bedtime.	d. Promotes comfort
_____ Always have William Jefferson void before going to bed.	e. Provides a mild sedative effect

Comfort

∽ **Reading Assignment:** Pain Management (Chapter 31)

Patients: Pablo Rodriguez, Medical-Surgical Floor, Room 405
Piya Jordan, Medical-Surgical Floor, Room 403

Objectives:

- Differentiate acute and chronic pain.
- Describe factors that influence pain.
- Identify presenting signs and symptoms of a patient in pain.
- Describe cultural implications in pain management.
- Apply critical thinking in the assessment of a patient in pain.
- Select appropriate pain relief interventions for patients in the case studies.
- Provide rationales for pain interventions as they apply to physiology of pain.
- Discuss principles for use of patient-controlled analgesia.
- Discuss implications for use of analgesics.
- Identify approaches for evaluating a patient's response to pain therapies.

Overview:

Pain is the most common reason why individuals seek health care. The experience of pain can affect an individual physically, psychologically, socially, and economically. Because pain is a subjective experience, it becomes critical for nurses to recognize that no painful event or experience is the same. A patient's personal experiences, values, and cultural background all influence the pain experience. You must respect a patient's perception and expression of pain and partner with the patient to find the most effective pain-relief strategies.

Comfort is a concept central to the art of nursing. Through comfort, nurses provide strength, hope, and assistance to clients. You must learn to combine pharmacologic and nonpharmacologic pain therapies to find the most effective approach to pain control. You are ethically and legally responsible for managing pain and relieving suffering. Effective pain management reduces physical discomfort and also improves a patient's quality of life.

Exercise 1

 CD-ROM Activity

 45 minutes

 In this exercise you will visit Pablo Rodriguez, a 71-year-old Hispanic male who is suffering from advanced non-small cell lung carcinoma. You may have worked with Pablo Rodriguez previously if you already completed Lesson 6, 11, 13, or 19.

- Sign in to work at Pacific View Regional Hospital on the Medical-Surgical Floor for Period of Care 1. (*Note:* If you are already in the virtual hospital from a previous exercise, click on **Leave the Floor** and then **Restart the Program** to get to the sign-in window.)
- From the Patient List, select Pablo Rodriguez (Room 405).
- Click on **Get Report**.
- Click on **Go to Nurses' Station**.
- Click on **Chart** and then on **405**.
- Click on and review the **Nursing Admission**.
- Click on and review the **History and Physical**.

1. Based on data from the Nursing Admission summary, list six different sources of discomfort that Pablo Rodriguez is experiencing.

2. Which of the following best describes the pain of the subcutaneous nodules?
   a. Neuropathic pain
   b. Acute pain
   c. Idiopathic pain
   d. Nociceptive somatic pain

3. Pablo Rodriguez is experiencing chronic pain. Indicate whether each of the following statements about chronic pain is true or false.

   a. _____   Chronic pain from cancer may be sensed at the actual site of the tumor or distant from the site.

   b. _____   Chronic pain commonly causes fatigue, anorexia, weight loss, and insomnia.

   c. _____   Chronic pain usually has a predictable ending.

   d. _____   A common problem in the management of chronic pain is under-treatment.

• Click on **Return to Nurses' Station** and then on **405** at the bottom of the screen.
- Review the **Initial Observations.**
- Click on **Patient Care** and then on **Nurse-Client Interactions**.
- Select and view the video titled **0730: Symptom Management**. (*Note:* Check the virtual clock to see whether enough time has elapsed. You can use the fast-forward feature to advance the time by 2-minute intervals if the video is not yet available. Then click again on **Patient Care** and **Nurse-Client Interactions** to refresh the screen.)

4. Name two factors identified in Pablo Rodriguez's admission data that would increase his perception of pain.

5. Pablo Rodriguez's Hispanic culture influences how he experiences pain and how he is able to express it with family and caregivers. In the nursing history, the patient reported that he wishes the pain to "go away." Based on your observation of the patient during the video, which of the following statements accurately describes factors the nurse should consider in his care? Select all that apply.

_____ The nurse may need to use probing questions to assess Pablo Rodriguez's pain thoroughly.

_____ The patient's feelings about the meaning of pain will affect his perception of it.

_____ Knowing the nature of cancer pain, the nurse should presume how Pablo Rodriguez will respond.

_____ Whether Pablo Rodriguez is stoic or expressive about pain reflects his Hispanic culture.

_____ Pablo Rodriguez's language barrier makes it difficult to assess his pain.

 • Click on **EPR** at the top of your screen; then click on **Login**.
- Specify **405** from the Patient drop-down menu and select **Vital Signs** from the Category drop-down menu.
- Review the pain assessment for Pablo Rodriguez.

6. From the following list, identify the characteristics that are included in the EPR assessment of Pablo Rodriguez's pain. Select all that apply.

_____ Pain location

_____ Pain intensity

_____ Pain onset

_____ Pain quality

_____ Behavioral effects

_____ Contributing factors

_____ Influence on activities of daily living

- Click on **Exit EPR.**
- Click on **Chart** and then **405.**
- Click on **Physician's Orders.**
- Review the orders for Tuesday at 2300.

7. The EPR data indicated that relieving factors could be referred to in the Physician's Orders. What is wrong with such an assessment finding?

8. The physician has ordered patient-controlled analgesia (PCA) with the following order: Morphine sulfate 0.5 mg IV every 10 min/12 mg in 4-hour lockout. Over a period of 1 hour, what would Pablo Rodriguez's maximal dose be?
   a. 10 mg
   b. 3 mg
   c. 30 mg
   d. 12 mg

9. If, in describing use of the PCA, Pablo Rodriguez said to you, "I am afraid to keep pushing this button so often," what would you say?

10. Morphine is an opiate. What complications does it cause that could worsen Pablo Rodriguez's current condition?

- Click on **Return to Room 405.**
- Click on **Leave the Floor.**
- Click on **Restart the Program.**
- Sign in to work at Pacific View Regional Hospital on the Medical-Surgical Floor for Period of Care 2.
- From the Patient List, select Pablo Rodriguez (Room 405).
- Click on **Get Report.**
- Click on **Go to Nurses' Station.**
- Click on **EPR.**
- Click on **Login.**
- Select **405** from the Patient drop-down menu and **Vital Signs** from the Category drop-down menu.

11. In a comparison of patient-controlled analgesia with continuous IV analgesic infusion, what is the advantage of continuous IV infusion?
    a. Allows patient to gain control over pain by accessing medication when needed
    b. Provides a local anesthetic, avoiding systemic effects of analgesia
    c. Avoids the serious sedative effects of parenteral narcotics
    d. Offers uniform pain control with fewer peaks and valleys in plasma analgesic concentration

 • Still in the EPR, review Pablo Rodriguez's pain assessments.

12. Record Pablo Rodriguez's pain intensity scores for the times specified in the chart below.

	Wed 0700	Wed 0730	Wed 0900	Wed 1000	Wed 1100
Pain Score					

13. What does the pattern of pain severity scores tell you about Pablo Rodriguez's pain control? What intervention would you recommend after seeing this pattern of data?

Exercise 2

 CD-ROM Activity

 30 minutes

 In this exercise you will visit Pablo Rodriguez, a 71-year-old Hispanic male who is suffering from advanced non-small cell lung carcinoma. You may have worked with Pablo Rodriguez previously if you already completed Exercise 1 of this lesson or Lesson 6, 11, 13, or 19.

• Sign in to work at Pacific View Regional Hospital on the Medical-Surgical Floor for Period of Care 2. (*Note:* If you are already in the virtual hospital from a previous exercise, click on **Leave the Floor** and then **Restart the Program** to get to the sign-in window.)
• From the Patient List, select Pablo Rodriguez (Room 405).
• Click on **Get Report** and then **Go to Nurses' Station**.
• Click on **Chart** and then on **405**.
• Click on and review the **Nursing Admission**.

1. Complete the following assessment form as you review Pablo Rodriguez's clinical summary and admission data.

Assessment Category	Relevant Data for Pablo Rodriguez
Age	
Activity/Rest	
Energy level	
Sleep quality	
Ability to perform ADLs	
Mobility limitations	
Nutrition	
Appetite	
Weight change	
Oral cavity abnormalities	
Nausea/vomiting?	
Comfort	
Pain severity	
Location	
Quality	
Alleviating factors	
Aggravating factors	
Self-Concept	

2. Pablo Rodriguez's data reveal a number of nursing diagnoses. Match the defining characteristics below with the four diagnoses that apply to the patient. Each defining characteristic may apply to more than one nursing diagnosis. (*Study Tip:* Refer to the NANDA international nursing diagnoses and defining characteristics listings.)

Nursing Diagnoses	Defining Characteristics
_____ Nausea	a. Experiencing metallic taste
_____ Chronic Pain	b. Pain reported as 5 on a scale of 0-to-10 scale
_____ Fatigue	c. Reports difficulty falling asleep
_____ Imbalanced Nutrition: Less Than Body Requirements	d. Unable to maintain usual routines
	e. Lost 50 pounds last year
	f. Reports feeling nauseated
	g. Reports feeling weak and tired
	h. Sore, inflamed gums
	i. Loss of appetite
	j. States, "I am a burden." Feels guilt in not meeting responsibilities

→ • Still in the chart, click on the **Patient Education** notes and review the information given.

3. Explain the purpose for educating the patient about mouth care.

4. Consider what you know about Pablo Rodriguez. Listed below and on the next page are nonpharmacologic pain-relief interventions that may or may not be appropriate in helping Pablo Rodriguez obtain pain relief. Provide a rationale to explain why or why not to use each of the therapies for Pablo Rodriguez at this time.

Progressive relaxation

Back rub

Removing pain stimuli

Music

5. Pablo Rodriguez reports that his pain is aggravated by pressure from positioning. What intervention might you try?

Exercise 3

 CD-ROM Activity

 30 minutes

 In this exercise you will visit Piya Jordan, a 68-year-old Asian-American female who entered the hospital after an emergency department admission for abdominal pain, nausea, and vomiting. She underwent abdominal surgery for the removal of a mass in her right lower quadrant. You may have worked with Piya Jordan previously if you already completed Lesson 7, 10, 14, or 15.

- Sign in to work at Pacific View Regional Hospital on the Medical-Surgical Floor for Period of Care 1. (*Note:* If you are already in the virtual hospital from a previous exercise, click on **Leave the Floor** and then **Restart the Program** to get to the sign-in window.)
- From the Patient List, select Piya Jordan (Room 403).
- Click on **Get Report**.
- Click on **Go to Nurses' Station**.
- Click on **Chart** and then on **403**.
- Click on and review the **History and Physical**.

1. After reviewing the History and Physical and the description of Piya Jordan's pain, how would you critique the quality of the physician's pain assessment? Explain.

 • Now review the **Nursing Admission**, specifically the Comfort section near the end of the data form.

2. What characteristics of pain are missing from the Nursing Admission description?

 • Click on **Return to Nurses' Station**.
- Click on **EPR**.
- Click on **Login**.
- Specify **403** from the Patient drop-down menu and **Vital Signs** from the Category drop-down menu.
- Review the pain assessment.

3. Based on the data from the EPR, Piya Jordan is experiencing acute postoperative incisional pain. Her clinical summary reported restlessness and confusion from an overdose of meperidine through her PCA. What would be the priority nursing measure to initiate?
   a. Increase the dosing interval for administration of meperidine.
   b. Initiate more frequent vital signs, including pain assessment.
   c. Reeducate Piya Jordan and her daughter about the proper way to self-administer PCA doses.
   d. Stop the PCA infusion and consult with the physician about changing the drug in the PCA and treating the patient for side effects.

 • Click on **Exit EPR** and then on **Return to Nurses' Station**.
- Click on **403** at the bottom of the screen to enter Piya Jordan's room.
- Review the **Initial Observations**.
- Click on **Patient Care** and then on **Nurse-Client Interactions**.
- Select and view the video titled **0735: Pain—Adverse Drug Event Interaction**. (*Note:* Check the virtual clock to see whether enough time has elapsed. You can use the fast-forward feature to advance the time by 2-minute intervals if the video is not yet available. Then click again on **Patient Care** and **Nurse-Client Interactions** to refresh the screen.)

4. Nonpharmacologic pain-relief interventions can be appropriate for patients in acute pain. What do you know about Piya Jordan that might make nonpharmacologic interventions appealing?

5. The Nursing Admission summary noted that Piya Jordan used a heating pad at home for pain relief. A heating pad provides pain relief through which action?
   a. Biofeedback
   b. Distraction
   c. Reducing pain perception
   d. Cutaneous stimulation

6. Piya Jordan was reported at 0700 to have confusion and restlessness. Would use of a heating pad have been appropriate for pain relief at that time? Explain.

7. Assume that a nurse assistant who is helping you care for Piya Jordan comes to you in the hallway and says, "The patient told me she is having pain. She said it was a 7." What should you do?
   a. Go to Piya Jordan and assess the severity and character of her pain and assess her wound.
   b. Prepare an analgesic and then go to Piya Jordan's room.
   c. Prepare an analgesic and notify the physician that the patient's pain has increased.
   d. Go to Piya Jordan and assess the severity and character of her pain.

LESSON 13 ——————————

Nutrition

∞ **Reading Assignment:** Nutrition (Chapter 32)

Patients: Jacquline Catanazaro, Medical-Surgical Floor, Room 402
Pablo Rodriguez, Medical-Surgical Floor, Room 405

Objectives:

- Compute a BMI for a patient in a case study.
- Identify the function of select nutrients.
- Describe factors that place patients at risk for nutritional problems.
- Conduct a dietary history.
- Identify clinical signs of nutritional alterations.
- Identify appropriate diet therapies for patients in the case studies.

Overview:

One of the basic needs that you as a nurse must provide your patients with is well-balanced, appropriate nutrition. Without adequate nutrition a patient will not have normal immune function or growth, proper wound healing or energy levels, or normal metabolic function. Many factors can affect a patient's willingness and ability to eat as a result of illness or injury. Thus it becomes your responsibility to know how physiologic alterations affect a patient's ability to take in and digest food, factors that alter the patient's appetite, and the effects of therapeutic diet regimens. Anticipating a patient's nutritional needs can be very effective in preventing many complications of disease. In some illnesses, such as type 1 diabetes mellitus or mild hypertension, diet therapy may be the major treatment for disease control. The patient must be an active partner in helping to select meal plans and approaches that will promote or enhance nutritional intake.

Exercise 1

 CD-ROM Activity

 30 minutes

 In this exercise you will visit Jacquline Catanazaro, a 45-year-old Caucasian female who has a 30-year history of asthma, complicated by schizophrenia. She has been admitted to the emergency department because of an acute asthma episode and concurrent schizophrenic episode. You may have worked with Jacquline Catanazaro previously if you already completed Lesson 9 or 14.

- Sign in to work at Pacific View Regional Hospital on the Medical-Surgical Floor for Period of Care 1. (*Note:* If you are already in the virtual hospital from a previous exercise, click on **Leave the Floor** and then **Restart the Program** to get to the sign-in window.)
- From the Patient List, select Jacquline Catanazaro (Room 402).
- Click on **Get Report**.
- Click on **Go to Nurses' Station**.
- Click on **Chart** and then on **402**.
- Click on and review the **Nursing Admission**.

1. Based on your review of the information in the Nursing Admission, complete the following dietary history.

History Component	Jacquline Catanazaro's Data
Height	
Weight	
History of food allergies	
Number of meals per day	
Food preferences	
Food preparation practices	
Appetite	
History of weight change	
Condition of oral cavity	
Bowel elimination	

2. Compute Jacquline Catanazaro's BMI. (*Study Tip:* There are 2.2 pounds in a kilogram; 1 meter equals 39.37 inches.)

3. Does Jacquline Catanazaro's BMI confirm the admission history report that the patient is obese?

→ • Click on and review the patient's **History and Physical**.
  • Review the **Consultations**, specifically the Psychiatric Consult.

4. Which of the following factors most likely has contributed to Jacquline Catanazaro's loss of appetite for the last week? Select all that apply.

_____ Albuterol

_____ Anxiety

_____ Loxapine

_____ Shortness of breath

_____ Excessive sleep

Fill in the blanks in the following statements regarding food nutrients.

5. _____ are the most calorie-dense nutrients.

6. The main source of energy in the diet is _____.

7. Based on the food guide pyramid in your textbook, Jacquline Catanazaro should eat

   _____ servings of vegetables daily.

8. A regular diet includes _____ restrictions.

9. Jacquline Catanazaro's constipation might be relieved by an increase in fruits, vegetables,

   and _____.

10. Once Jacquline Catanazaro is discharged, what would be an appropriate approach for assessing her nutritional intake?

11. Based on your review of the patient's medical record, list three interventions you might use to improve Jacquline Catanazaro's nutritional status.

Exercise 2

 CD-ROM Activity

 30 minutes

In this exercise you will visit Pablo Rodriguez, a 71-year-old Hispanic male who is suffering from advanced-stage lung cancer. You may have worked with Pablo Rodriguez previously if you already completed Lesson 6, 11, 12, or 19.

- Sign in to work at Pacific View Regional Hospital on the Medical-Surgical Floor for Period of Care 2. (*Note:* If you are already in the virtual hospital from a previous exercise, click on **Leave the Floor** and then **Restart the Program** to get to the sign-in window.)
- From the Patient List, select Pablo Rodriguez (Room 405).
- Click on **Get Report**.
- Click on **Go to Nurses' Station**.
- Click on **Chart** and then on **405**.
- Click on and review the **Nursing Admission**.
- Click on and review the **History and Physical**.

1. List three factors that may contribute to Pablo Rodriguez's loss of appetite.

2. Match each nursing diagnosis with its cluster of defining characteristics.

Nursing Diagnosis	Defining Characteristic Cluster
_____ Nausea	a. Sore buccal cavity, aversion to eating, body weight 20% below ideal, poor muscle tone
_____ Imbalanced Nutrition: Less Than Body Requirements	b. Metallic taste, aversion to food, reports feeling of nausea
_____ Chronic Pain	c. Weight change, changes in sleep pattern, fatigue, loss of appetite

3. Is Pablo Rodriguez a candidate for enteral feeding? Explain.

4. Pablo Rodriguez has received chemotherapy and radiation, both of which can affect a patient's immune system. His loss of 50 lb over a year and his current symptoms indicate malnutrition. Malnutrition can cause which of the following?
   a. Increased skin density
   b. Shorter time for activation of lymphocytes
   c. Reduced antibodies
   d. Increased T cell formation

5. Based on your chart review, which of the following physical findings could be related to Pablo Rodriguez's nutritional status? Select all that apply.

   _____ Mild swelling of lower extremities

   _____ Skin warm and dry

   _____ No accessory muscle use

   _____ Swollen red gums

   _____ Capillary refill greater than 4 seconds

   _____ General muscle weakness

6. Assume that you have been successful in controlling Pablo Rodriguez's nausea and vomiting. Describe three approaches you could use to improve his appetite.

Elimination

✐ **Reading Assignment:** Urinary Elimination (Chapter 33)
Bowel Elimination (Chapter 34)

Patients: Piya Jordan, Medical-Surgical Floor, Room 403
Jacquline Catanazaro, Medical-Surgical Floor, Room 402

Objectives:

- Describe factors that influence normal defecation.
- Describe factors that influence normal urination.
- Collect a nursing history of a patient's elimination status in a case study.
- Develop a plan of care for a patient with a bowel elimination alteration.
- Identify nursing interventions used to manage bowel elimination problems.
- Describe principles used in the care of an indwelling urinary catheter.
- Describe nursing interventions designed to reduce the risk for urinary tract infection.

Overview:

Normal elimination of fecal and urinary wastes is essential for good health. When the urinary system fails to function normally, all body systems can become affected. Alterations in bowel elimination are often early signs and symptoms of problems within the gastrointestinal or other body systems. In addition, patients may experience emotional upset from having elimination alterations.

Elimination patterns and habits vary among individuals. Thus, as a nurse, you must assess any elimination problems thoroughly while applying knowledge of anatomy and physiology of the urinary and bowel systems. Thoughtful critical thinking will allow you to identify patients' problems accurately and to select relevant nursing interventions.

Exercise 1

 CD-ROM Activity

 60 minutes

 In this exercise you will visit Piya Jordan, a 68-year-old Asian-American female who entered the hospital after an emergency department admission for abdominal pain, nausea, and vomiting. She underwent abdominal surgery for the removal of a mass in her right lower quadrant. You may have worked with Piya Jordan previously if you already completed Lesson 7, 10, 12, or 15.

- Sign in to work at Pacific View Regional Hospital on the Medical-Surgical Floor for Period of Care 1. (*Note:* If you are already in the virtual hospital from a previous exercise, click on **Leave the Floor** and then **Restart the Program** to get to the sign-in window.)
- From the Patient List, select Piya Jordan (Room 403).
- Click on **Get Report**.
- Click on **Go to Nurses' Station**.
- Click on **Chart** and then on **403**.
- Click on and review the **History and Physical**.
- Click on **Diagnostic Reports** and review the summary of the abdominal CT.
- Next, click on and review the **Physician's Notes**.

1. Piya Jordan's History & Physical reports that she had ribbonlike stool and blood. Explain the source of these symptoms.

2. Based on your review of the abdominal CT summary, removal of Piya Jordan's mass would likely cause what change in her elimination in the future? Explain.

 • Click on and review the **Nursing Admission**.

3. As you review Piya Jordan's admission data, complete the nursing history form below.

Nursing History Summary

Usual urinary elimination pattern

Symptoms of urinary alteration

Normal fluid intake

History of urinary problems

Usual bowel elimination pattern

Symptoms of bowel elimination alteration

Physical findings

Exercise pattern

Diet history

Able to toilet independently?

---

4. Match each of the following factors with its corresponding effect on bowel elimination.

Factor	Effect on Bowel Elimination
_____ Physical activity	a. Increases peristalsis
_____ Fluid intake less than 1000 mL daily	b. Decreases peristalsis
_____ High-fiber diet	c. Suppresses defecation
_____ Older adulthood	
_____ Pain	
_____ Lactose intolerance	

5. Based on your knowledge that Piya Jordan has had a colon resection, as well as your review of her elimination history, list three recommendations you would make to her to ensure normal bowel elimination once she goes home.

 • Still in the chart, review the **Physician's Orders**.

6. Piya Jordan has had a urinalysis ordered for which of the following reasons?
   a. It is needed as a preoperative screening.
   b. Her intravenous infusion contains potassium.
   c. Her past history of diabetes mellitus suggests glucose may be in urine.
   d. She is at risk for infection because of the presence of the urinary catheter.

7. Piya Jordan has a history of stress incontinence and urgency. For each of the interventions listed below, provide a rationale.

Intervention	Rationale
Before discharge, have patient practice how to perform pelvic floor exercises	
Initiate a toilet schedule on awakening	
Minimize the intake of tea and cola	
Practice deep breathing and have patient read when voiding	

8. Piya Jordan has a urinary catheter in place. List several sites where infectious organisms might enter a urinary drainage system.

 • Click on **Return to Nurses' Station**.
 • Click on **403** at the bottom of the screen.
 • Review the **Initial Observations**.
 • Click on **Patient Care** and then on **Physical Assessment**.

9. In the left column below, list the physical assessment categories you would select to perform a focused assessment of the function and effects of Piya Jordan's urinary catheter. For each category, provide a rationale for your selection.

Categories to Assess   **Rationale**

 • Based on your answer to question 9, perform the focused assessment on Piya Jordan by clicking on the appropriate categories and subcategories.

10. During the pelvic examination, the urologic assessment included a photo of Piya Jordan's catheter and drainage system. Was the catheter and drainage system anchored and positioned correctly? Explain.

11. For each of the following outcomes resulting from urinary catheterization, identify the intervention you would provide.

Outcome	Intervention
Urine drains freely, clear yellow	
Patient develops fever; urine has a foul odor	
Patient complains of perineal irritation at urethra	
Patient denies bladder discomfort	

Exercise 2

 CD-ROM Activity

 30 minutes

 In this exercise you will meet Jacquline Catanazaro, a 45-year-old Caucasian female with a 30-year history of asthma, complicated by schizophrenia. She has been admitted to the ED because of an acute asthma episode and concurrent schizophrenic episode. You may have worked with Jacquline Catanazaro previously if you completed Lesson 9 or 13.

- Sign in to work at Pacific View Regional Hospital on the Medical-Surgical Floor for Period of Care 2. (*Note:* If you are already in the virtual hospital from a previous exercise, click on **Leave the Floor** and then **Restart the Program** to get to the sign-in window.)
- From the Patient List, select Jacquline Catanazaro (Room 402).
- Click on **Get Report**.
- Click on **Go to Nurses' Station**.
- Click on **Chart** and then on **402**.
- Click on **Nursing Admission** and review.

1. Which of the following factors contribute to Jacquline Catanazaro's bowel elimination problems? Select all that apply.

_____ Physical inactivity

_____ Age

_____ Emotional stress

_____ Limited intake of high-fiber foods

_____ Reduced fluid intake

_____ Obesity

2. Jacquline Catanazaro's Nursing Admission states that she reports a pattern of a bowel movement every 1 to 2 days and perceives having constipation. She also reports a hard stool. What two additional symptoms might you assess to confirm constipation for this patient?

• Click on **Return to Nurses' Station**.
• Click on **402** at the bottom of the screen to enter the patient's room.
• Review the **Initial Observations**.
• Click on **Patient Care** and then on **Physical Assessment**.
• Click on **Abdomen** and review the examination of the abdomen.

3. Listed below are physical findings that Jacquline Catanazaro has exhibited. Next to each finding, describe what you would more likely find if the patient had constipation instead.

Physical Finding	Constipation Finding
Abdomen soft and flat	
Bowel sounds normal	
No abdominal tenderness or masses	

• Click on **Patient Care** and then on **Nurse-Client Interactions**.
• Select and view the video titled **1140: Compliance—Medications**. (*Note:* Check the virtual clock to see whether enough time has elapsed. You can use the fast-forward feature to advance the time by 2-minute intervals if the video is not yet available. Then click again on **Patient Care** and **Nurse-Client Interactions** to refresh the screen.)

4. Jacquline Catanazaro's Nursing Admission and the video reveal the three data clusters listed below. For each cluster, identify the appropriate nursing diagnosis. (*Study Tip:* Refer to a resource for NANDA nursing diagnoses.)

Data Cluster	Nursing Diagnosis
Emotional stress Insufficient fiber intake Poor eating habits; does not eat vegetables or fruits Insufficient fluid intake Antipsychotic/sedative use	
Dysfunctional eating pattern, 4 to 6 meals a day Sedentary activity level Weight 20% over ideal for height	

Inability to take responsibility for
  meeting health practices; does
  not remember to take medications
Lack of adaptive behavior to
  environmental changes; anxious
  and agitated
Lack of knowledge regarding health
  practices; "It takes a lot for me to
  remember"	

5. Consider how the nursing diagnoses you identified in question 4 are interrelated. Below, develop a plan of care for the nursing diagnosis Risk for Constipation.

Plan of Care Component

Goal

Outcomes

Interventions

Rationales

6. Assume that the nurse was to consult with the physician about ordering a medication for Jacquline Catanazaro. What might be the best recommendation to relieve her constipation? Explain.

7. If you were the nurse caring for Jacquline Catanazaro 2 days after initiating treatment for constipation, what evaluation measures would you use to determine whether the plan of care was effective?

Care of the Surgical Patient

Reading Assignment: Skin Integrity and Wound Care (Chapter 36)
Surgical Patient (Chapter 38)

Patient: Piya Jordan, Medical-Surgical Floor, Room 403

Objectives:

- Describe criteria to use in the preoperative assessment of a surgical patient.
- Explain the rationale for postoperative exercises.
- Discuss principles to incorporate in a preoperative teaching plan.
- Describe risks for postoperative complications in case study patients.
- Identify risks associated with different forms of anesthesia.
- Apply critical thinking to the assessment of a postoperative patient.
- Identify signs and symptoms of common postoperative complications.
- Describe nursing interventions for preventing postoperative complications.

Overview:

Perioperative nursing care is the care administered before (preoperative), during (intraoperative), and after (postoperative) surgery. Because surgery occurs in both outpatient and inpatient settings, a surgical nurse must be able to anticipate patients' risks for problems, know the anticipated effects of surgery, recognize early signs of complications, and know how to intervene in all situations. Patients who undergo surgery become dependent on the nurse for physical as well as psychological comfort. However, when patients become active participants in their preoperative and postoperative care, the incidence of complications is less likely. Thorough preoperative education is essential to ensure appropriate and safe care for the surgical patient.

Exercise 1

 CD-ROM Activity

 45 minutes

In this exercise you will visit Piya Jordan, a 68-year-old Asian-American female who entered the hospital after an emergency department admission for abdominal pain, nausea, and vomiting. She underwent abdominal surgery for the removal of a mass in her right lower quadrant. You may have worked with Piya Jordan previously if you already completed Lesson 7, 10, 12, or 14.

- Sign in to work at Pacific View Regional Hospital on the Medical-Surgical Floor for Period of Care 1. (*Note:* If you are already in the virtual hospital from a previous exercise, click on **Leave the Floor** and then **Restart the Program** to get to the sign-in window.)
- From the Patient List, select Piya Jordan (Room 403).
- Click on **Get Report**.
- Click on **Go to Nurses' Station**.
- Click on **Chart** and then on **403**.
- Review the **Nursing Admission**.

1. Based on the Nursing Admission data, identify which of the surgical risk factors apply to Piya Jordan. Select all that apply.

_____ Obesity

_____ Heart disease

_____ Fever

_____ Nutritional imbalance

_____ Chronic pain

_____ Age

_____ Liver disease

2. Identify two alterations of the cardiovascular system that may apply to Piya Jordan because of her age.

- Click on and review the **History and Physical**.
- Click on and review the **Laboratory Results**.

3. The physician's History and Physical noted the need to correct Piya Jordan's electrolytes and reverse anticoagulation before surgery. Which laboratory values were abnormal in Piya Jordan's case? Select all that apply.

_____ RBC

_____ INR

_____ Potassium

_____ Sodium

_____ Hgb

_____ Creatinine

4. Explain why you think Piya Jordan's Hgb and RBC values were lower than normal before surgery. Why are changes in these lab values significant?

5. What is the most likely reason that Piya Jordan's INR is higher than normal?
   a. Inflammation of her knee joints
   b. Warfarin therapy at home
   c. Irregular nature of her heart rate
   d. Blood in her stool

6. Because of the elevated INR, Piya Jordan would be at risk for which of the following complications during surgery?
   a. Urinary retention
   b. Pneumonia
   c. Paralytic ileus
   d. Hemorrhage

 • Still in the chart, click again on **Nursing Admission** and review the summaries for Perception and Cognition, Self-Perception, Role Relationships, and Coping and Stress Tolerance.

 • Now click on **Nurse's Notes** and review the notes from Tuesday 0330 to Tuesday 0900.

7. The nurse's assessment should focus on factors that will influence the ability to provide Piya Jordan with preoperative instruction. Listed below are numerous factors identified in Piya Jordan's assessment. Complete this exercise by indicating whether each factor would facilitate instruction (positive) or would be a barrier to instruction (negative).

Assessment Factor	Effect on Instruction
_____ Patient reports a pain score of 8 out of 10.	a. Positive
_____ Patient expresses being anxious about husband's welfare.	b. Negative
_____ Daughter is supportive of mother.	
_____ Patient is fearful of cancer diagnosis.	
_____ Patient speaks English and has college education.	
_____ Patient reports feeling nauseated.	

8. Based on information from the Nurse's Notes and Nursing Admission, what would be the best time to teach Piya Jordan about deep breathing and coughing exercises? Give a rationale.

9. After surgery, it is important to turn patients frequently. What factor in Piya Jordan's history might make turning difficult for her?

10. Match each preoperative exercise listed below with the postoperative complication(s) the exercise prevents. Each exercise can have more than one answer.

Preoperative Exercise	Postoperative Complication
_____ Deep breathing	a. Pneumonia
_____ Coughing	b. Thrombus formation
_____ Turning	c. Atelectasis
_____ Leg exercises	d. Joint immobility
_____ Incentive spirometry	

Exercise 2

 CD-ROM Activity

 30 minutes

 In this exercise you will visit Piya Jordan, a 68-year-old Asian-American female who entered the hospital after an emergency department admission for abdominal pain, nausea, and vomiting. She underwent abdominal surgery for the removal of a mass in her right lower quadrant. You may have worked with Piya Jordan previously if you already completed Exercise 1 of this lesson or Lesson 7, 10, 12, or 14.

• Sign in to work at Pacific View Regional Hospital on the Medical-Surgical Floor for Period of Care 1. (*Note:* If you are already in the virtual hospital from a previous exercise, click on **Leave the Floor** and then **Restart the Program** to get to the sign-in window.)
• From the Patient List, select Piya Jordan (Room 403).
• Click on **Get Report**.
• Click on **Go to Nurses' Station**.
• Click on **Chart** and then on **403**.
• Click on and review the **Nurse's Notes**.
• Next, review the **Postoperative Notes**.
• Finally, review the **Physician's Notes**.

1. For each of the interventions listed below and on the next page, give a rationale for its use in Piya Jordan's case.

Jackson-Pratt drain

Sequential compression device

Nasogastric tube

Abdominal dressing

2. Which of the following findings is abnormal in Piya Jordan's case?
   a. Nasogastric tube draining moderate brown drainage
   b. Telemetry showing atrial fibrillation
   c. Urine clear, dark yellow
   d. Jackson-Pratt draining serosanguinous drainage

3. After reviewing the clinical summary and the Nurse's Notes, what common postoperative complication might Piya Jordan be at risk for, unless the nurse actively intervenes? Give a rationale and explain the interventions required.

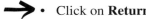 • Click on **Return to Nurses' Station**.
   • Select **403** at the bottom of the screen.
   • Click on **Patient Care** and then on **Physical Assessment**.
   • Click on **Abdomen**.
   • Review the findings of the abdominal assessment, specifically the subcategories of **Integumentary** and **Gastrointestinal**.

4. What type of dressing does Piya Jordan have over her abdomen? How is it secured?

5. What is the most critical time for healing of a surgical wound?
   a. First 24 hours postoperatively
   b. 7 days postoperatively
   c. 24 to 72 hours postoperatively
   d. 15 to 20 days postoperatively

• Conduct a focused physical examination of Piya Jordan by clicking on the various yellow assessment buttons and green subcategories as needed based on your answer to question 6.

6. As the nurse caring for Piya Jordan postoperatively, you would want to do a focused assessment when you begin your care. Which assessment categories would you select to focus on her postoperative status? (*Hint:* Do not forget to assess equipment.)

 • When you have completed your focused assessment, click on **Leave the Floor**.
• From the Floor Menu, choose **Look at Your Preceptor's Evaluation**.
• Next, click on **Examination Report** to see how you did.
• Click on **Return to Evaluations**.
• Click on **Return to Menu**.

Exercise 3

 CD-ROM Activity

 45 minutes

 In this exercise you will visit Piya Jordan, a 68-year-old Asian-American female who entered the hospital after an emergency department admission for abdominal pain, nausea, and vomiting. She underwent abdominal surgery for the removal of a mass in her right lower quadrant. You may have worked with Piya Jordan previously if you already completed Exercise 1 or 2 of this lesson or Lesson 7, 10, 12, or 14.

• Sign in to work at Pacific View Regional Hospital on the Medical-Surgical Floor for Period of Care 2. (*Note:* If you are already in the virtual hospital from a previous exercise, click on **Leave the Floor** and then **Restart the Program** to get to the sign-in window.)
• From the Patient List, select Piya Jordan (Room 403).
• Click on **Get Report**.
• Click on **Go to Nurses' Station**.
• Click on **Chart** and then on **403**.
• Click on and review the **Nursing Admission**.
• Click on and review the **Surgical Reports**.

1. Considering the type of anesthesia Piya Jordan received, she is most at risk for which of the following?
   a. Respiratory depression, cardiovascular irritability, and liver damage
   b. Respiratory paralysis and hypotension
   c. Loss of sensation and pain reception in operative area
   d. Headache, urinary retention, and back pain

 • Click on **Nurse's Notes** and review the notes for Wednesday at 1115.
   • Click on **Return to Nurses' Station**.
   • Select **403** at the bottom of the screen.
   • Review the **Initial Observations**.
   • Click on **Patient Care** and then **Nurse-Client Interactions**.
   • Select and view the video titled **1115: Interventions—Nausea, Blood**. (*Note:* Check the virtual clock to see whether enough time has elapsed. You can use the fast-forward feature to advance the time by 2-minute intervals if the video is not yet available. Then click again on **Patient Care** and **Nurse-Client Interactions** to refresh the screen.)

2. Piya Jordan is complaining of nausea. What is the likely source of the nausea?

3. Identify three assessments necessary to determine the source and nature of Piya Jordan's nausea.

4. When a nasogastric tube's patency is in question, what is the appropriate action?
   a. Remove the tube from suction and call the physician.
   b. Irrigate the tube with normal saline.
   c. Reposition the tube.
   d. Obtain an x-ray of the abdomen.

 • Click on **Physical Assessment**.
   • Click on **Chest** and then on the appropriate subcategories to review the assessment of Piya Jordan's chest.
   • Next, click on **Abdomen** and the related subcategories to review the abdominal assessment.
   • Now click on **Take Vital Signs** at the top of the screen.

5. From a review of the available findings for Piya Jordan, clusters of data can be formed. One data cluster for this patient is listed below.

   - Chest expansion decreased
   - Decreased aeration, both lower lobes
   - Acute pain
   - Abdomen tender to palpation
   - Has not used incentive spirometer

   What potential problem/nursing diagnosis is indicated by this data cluster?

6. A nurse who has cared for Piya Jordan tells you that one of her nursing diagnoses is Risk for Infection. Give a rationale for why this diagnosis would apply to Piya Jordan.

7. Below, complete the plan of care for the nursing diagnosis Ineffective Breathing Pattern.

Plan of Care Component

Goal

Expected Outcomes

Interventions

1.

2.

3.

4.

Evaluation Measures

1.

2.

3.

Wound Care

👓 **Reading Assignment:** Health Assessment and Physical Examination (Chapter 15)
Skin Integrity and Wound Care (Chapter 36)

Patients: Harry George, Medical-Surgical Floor, Room 401
Goro Oishi, Skilled Nursing Floor, Room 505

Objectives:

- Describe risk factors contributing to pressure ulcer formation.
- Use a pressure ulcer risk assessment tool for a patient in a case study.
- Explain factors that slow or promote wound healing.
- Identify types of wounds.
- Describe characteristics of a wound.
- Identify interventions used in the prevention of pressure ulcers.
- Explain the purpose of a wound dressing.
- Discuss factors to consider in selecting a wound dressing.
- Describe steps used in the application of dressings.

Overview:

The skin is a protective barrier against disease-causing organisms, and it is a sensory organ for pain, temperature, and touch. A break in skin integrity resulting from pressure, trauma, or surgical intervention creates a risk for patients, especially those with impaired wound healing. Good wound care practices involve active prevention. For example, a patient at risk for developing a pressure ulcer should be routinely mobilized or repositioned and given the appropriate type of skin care. A patient with a surgical wound requires meticulous wound care to prevent infection. As a nurse, you should know the risks associated with skin breakdown and the normal processes of wound healing to enable you to provide safe and appropriate care to your patients.

Exercise 1

 CD-ROM Activity

 45 minutes

 In this exercise you will visit Harry George, a 54-year-old Caucasian male who was admitted to the hospital with symptoms of infection and swelling of the foot. He has a history of abusing alcohol. He has been diagnosed with cellulitis and osteomyelitis of the foot. You may have worked with Harry George previously if you already completed Lesson 1, 17, or 18.

• Sign in to work at Pacific View Regional Hospital on the Medical-Surgical Floor for Period of Care 1. (*Note:* If you are already in the virtual hospital from a previous exercise, click on **Leave the Floor** and then **Restart the Program** to get to the sign-in window.)
• From the Patient List, select Harry George (Room 401).
• Click on **Get Report**.
• Click on **Go to Nurses' Station**.
• Click on **Chart** and then on **401**.
• Click on and review the **Nursing Admission**.
• Next, click on and review the **History and Physical**.

1. Listed below are factors that influence wound healing. Identify which of the factors apply to Harry George. Select all that apply.

_____ Nutrition

_____ Smoking

_____ Circulation

_____ Drugs

_____ Obesity

_____ Infection

_____ Age

_____ Wound stress

_____ Diabetes

2. Explain how each of the following factors affects wound healing.

Circulation

Diabetes

Smoking

3. When providing care to Harry George, the nurse recognizes the need to include _____ g of protein to his daily diet to promote wound healing.
   a. 33
   b. 43
   c. 53
   d. 63

4. Based on the description of Harry George's wound, the type of drainage can best be described as:
   a. thick, yellow or brown.
   b. clear, watery plasma.
   c. pale, red, watery.
   d. bright red.

→ • Click on **Return to Nurses' Station**.
   • Click on **401** at the bottom of the screen.
   • Read the **Initial Observations** of Harry George's status.

5. Explain why Harry George's left foot is elevated.

→ • Next, click on **Patient Care** and then on **Physical Assessment**.
   • Select **Lower Extremities** and review each of the four subcategories for assessment findings.

6. Good wound assessment requires the use of appropriate physical assessment techniques. Match each physical assessment finding listed below with its correct assessment technique. (*Study Tip:* Review Chapter 15 in your textbook for techniques.)

Physical Finding	**Assessment Technique**
_____ Wound draining serous drainage	a. Inspection
_____ Posterior tibial pulse 1+ on left	b. Palpation
_____ Skin warm and dry	c. Measurement
_____ Open lesion 2-3 centimeters	
_____ Capillary refill sluggish	
_____ Erythema over anterior tibia	

7. What stage would you use to describe Harry George's wound?

- Click on **Chart** and then on **401**.
- Click on **History and Physical** and review, specifically the Social History section.

8. What factor(s) in Harry George's social history may be implicated in his ability to care for his wound? Explain.

- Now review the **Physician's Notes**.
- Next, click on **Consultations** and review the Wound Care Team summary note.

9. The wound care note describes Harry George's dressing as occlusive. Which of the following dressings is most likely being used for Harry George?
   a. Wet-to-dry
   b. Telfa gauze
   c. Hydrocolloid
   d. Foam dressing

10. Give a rationale for your answer to question 9.

11. List three nursing actions that are important when preparing a patient for a dressing change.

12. Indicate whether each of the following statements is true or false.

a. _____ Hydrocolloid dressings support wound healing by debriding necrotic wounds.

b. _____ Hydrogel dressings can absorb large amounts of exudate.

c. _____ Before removing a wet-to-dry dressing, you should moisten the dressing with saline.

d. _____ When selecting a dressing, you should choose one that keeps the surrounding intact skin dry.

Exercise 2

CD-ROM Activity

45 minutes

In this exercise you will visit Goro Oishi, a 66-year-old Asian-American male who is admitted for hospice care following an intracerebral hemorrhage. You may have worked with Goro Oishi previously if you already completed Lesson 8 or 17.

- Sign in to work at Pacific View Regional Hospital on the Skilled Nursing Floor for Period of Care 1. (*Note:* If you are already in the virtual hospital from a previous exercise, click on **Leave the Floor** and then **Restart the Program** to get to the sign-in window.)
- From the Patient List, select Goro Oishi (Room 505).
- Click on **Get Report**.
- Click on **Go to Nurses' Station**.
- Click on **Chart** and then on **505**.
- Review the **Nursing Admission**.

1. Which of the following risk factors does Goro Oishi have for developing a pressure ulcer. Select all that apply.

_____ Impaired sensation

_____ Impaired mobility

_____ Altered level of consciousness

_____ Moisture

2. What would be Goro Oishi's Braden Scale score? (*Study Tip:* Review pages 1079 through 1080 in your textbook.)

3. What intervention is most likely preventing prolonged exposure of Goro Oishi's skin to moisture?

 • Click on **Return to Nurses' Station**.
• Click on **505** at the bottom of the screen to enter Goro Oishi's room.
• Review the **Initial Observations**.
• Click on **Patient Care** and then on **Physical Assessment**.
• Review the assessment of the integument for each of the physical assessment categories. (*Study Tip:* First click on **Head & Neck** and select **Integumentary** from the list of subcategories. Next, click on **Chest** and then on **Integumentary**. Continue until you have reviewed the Integumentary assessments in all seven body areas.)

4. For Goro Oishi, list several areas where a pressure ulcer is at risk for developing.

 • Click on **EPR** and then on **Login**.
• Specify **505** from the Patient drop-down menu and **Integumentary** from the Category drop-down menu.
• Review the flow sheet data for the integument.
• Now select **Hygiene and Comfort** from the Category drop-down menu and review this flow sheet.

5. Goro Oishi's Braden Scale score indicates that he is at high risk for a pressure ulcer to develop. List three interventions for a high-risk ulcer prevention protocol.

6. Answer the following questions based on your review of the EPR data.

    a. Do you believe Goro Oishi is being turned often enough?

    b. What time is he due to be turned again on the current schedule?

    c. In what position should he be placed?

    d. What specialty mattress is currently in use?

7. Which of the following are correct interventions the nurse should perform each time Goro Oishi is turned? Select all that apply.

    _____ Assess the area the patient was previously lying over for redness.

    _____ Massage any area of redness.

    _____ Check underlying linen for moisture.

    _____ Apply additional moisturizer to the skin.

8. If you were selecting a support surface on which to place Goro Oishi, what type would you choose? Give a rationale.

→ • Click on **Exit EPR**.
   • Click on **Chart** and then on **505**.
   • Review the **Nurse's Notes**.

9. Goro Oishi is currently receiving IV fluids. The change in nutritional therapy recommended by the physician will provide what benefit?

LESSON **17** ——————————————————

Loss and Grief and Nursing Interventions to Support Coping

————————————————————————————

> **Reading Assignment:** Stress and Coping (Chapter 24)
> Loss and Grief (Chapter 25)

Patients: Goro Oishi, Skilled Nursing Floor, Room 505
Harry George, Medical-Surgical Floor, Room 401

Objectives:

- Describe types of loss.
- Describe loss and grief responses of patients and families in the case studies.
- Identify characteristics of a person experiencing grief.
- Explain the relationship between loss and stress.
- Describe coping mechanisms used by patients in the case studies.
- Describe the use of hope in support of a patient in grief.
- Describe principles of palliative care.
- Identify nursing diagnoses applicable to a patient requiring palliative care.
- Develop a concept map for a patient facing death.

Overview:

Loss and grief are experiences that affect patients, families, and caregivers alike. You probably entered the nursing profession to help patients recover from illness or to achieve an improved level of health. Your knowledge, experience, and skill cannot always result in a cure for your patients.

Patients and their families can experience loss and grief in many forms. It is important for a patient to be able to experience and express grief in order to achieve healing. As a nurse, you are responsible for helping patients feel and express their loss and find realistic and relevant ways of coping. In cases where patients face long-term chronic or terminal illness, palliative care becomes essential. Palliative care includes preventive and supportive interventions designed to help patients approach the end of their lives. Understanding grief and loss, the concepts of coping, and the principles of palliative care will prepare you to give skilled and compassionate care to those patients who face loss and death.

Exercise 1

 CD-ROM Activity

 60 minutes

In this exercise you will visit Goro Oishi, a 66-year-old Asian-American male who is admitted for hospice care following an intracerebral hemorrhage. You may have worked with Goro Oishi previously if you already completed Lesson 8 or 16.

- Sign in to work at Pacific View Regional Hospital on the Skilled Nursing Floor for Period of Care 1. (*Note:* If you are already in the virtual hospital from a previous exercise, click on **Leave the Floor** and then **Restart the Program** to get to the sign-in window.)
- From the Patient List, select Goro Oishi (Room 505).
- Click on **Get Report**.
- Click on **Go to Nurses' Station**.
- Click on **Chart** and then on **505**.
- Review the **Nursing Admission**.

1. Goro Oishi has been admitted for hospice care. Which of the following describe the components or features of a hospice care program? Select all that apply.

   _____ A facility for treatment of terminal illnesses

   _____ Treatment philosophy focused on symptom control

   _____ Interdisciplinary care team approach

   _____ Care providers setting goals made to meet the family's desires

   _____ Coordination of home care services

2. Patients experience different types of loss.

   a. Based on the Nursing Admission summary of Role Relationships, identify the type of loss Goro Oishi experienced just before his stroke. Explain the significance of this loss.

   b. How did Goro Oishi choose to cope with his loss?

• Click on and review the **Physician's Notes**.
   • Next, click on and review the **Nurse's Notes**.

3. The notes state that Goro Oishi's family feels conflicted about whether or not to initiate enteral feeding. Which of the stages of grief below might describe the family's response? Select all that apply.

_____ Adjusting to the environment without the deceased

_____ Reorganization

_____ Denial

_____ Bargaining

_____ Emotionally relocating the deceased

 • Click on **Return to Nurses' Station**.
   • Click on **505** at the bottom of the screen.
   • Read the **Initial Observations**.
   • Click on **Patient Care** and then on **Nurse-Client Interactions**.
   • Observe the following three video interactions: **0735: Assessment—Family, 0750: Family Conflict—Plan of Care**, and **0755: Death—The Right to Die**. (*Note:* Check the virtual clock to see whether enough time has elapsed. You can use the fast-forward feature to advance the time by 2-minute intervals if the video is not yet available. Then click again on **Patient Care** and **Nurse-Client Interactions** to refresh the screen.)

4. After considering data from the Nursing Admission and observing Goro Oishi's wife during the videos, you recognize a variety of factors influencing her perception of loss. For each of the following factors, describe the conditions affecting Mrs. Oishi's response to loss.

Nature of loss

Personal relationship

Culture

Spiritual belief

➡ • Click on **Physical Assessment**.
   • Review each of the physical examination categories.

5. As you review the physical examination, also consider data from the Nursing Admission. The data you obtain begin to form patterns of information. A patient in need of palliative care has numerous health problems. Summarize your findings for each category listed below.

Skin integrity

Mobility

Respirations

Airway status

Fluid balance

6. As you begin to see patterns in Goro Oishi's data, nursing diagnoses also begin to emerge. For each nursing diagnosis below, select the defining characteristic that best supports it.

<table>
<tr><td>Nursing Diagnosis</td><td>Defining Characteristic</td></tr>
<tr><td>_____ Impaired Bed Mobility</td><td>a. No gag reflex</td></tr>
<tr><td>_____ Risk for Aspiration</td><td>b. Cool and pale skin</td></tr>
<tr><td>_____ Risk for Impaired Skin Integrity</td><td>c. No spontaneous movement</td></tr>
<tr><td>_____ Impaired Gas Exchange</td><td>d. Shallow respirations</td></tr>
<tr><td></td><td>e. Unable to move limbs independently</td></tr>
<tr><td></td><td>f. Febrile</td></tr>
<tr><td></td><td>g. Unable to swallow</td></tr>
<tr><td></td><td>h. Physically immobile</td></tr>
<tr><td></td><td>i. Oxygen saturation 88%</td></tr>
</table>

- Click on **Leave the Floor**; then click on **Restart the Program**.
- Sign in to work on the Skilled Nursing Floor, this time for Period of Care 3.
- From the Patient List, select Goro Oishi (Room 505).
- Click on **Get Report** and review. Then click on **Go to Nurses' Station**.
- Click on **505** at bottom of the screen.
- Review the **Initial Observations**.
- Now click on **Patient Care** and then on **Nurse-Client Interactions**.
- Select and view the video titled **1500: Patient Decline**. (*Note:* Check the virtual clock to see whether enough time has elapsed. You can use the fast-forward feature to advance the time by 2-minute intervals if the video is not yet available. Then click again on **Patient Care** and **Nurse-Client Interactions** to refresh the screen.)

7. Goro Oishi is progressively worsening. His breathing pattern is becoming more dyspneic as intracranial pressure builds from his hemorrhage. List three approaches you can use to promote comfort for a patient with ineffective breathing patterns.

8. In the video interaction, the nurse asks Mrs. Oishi to leave the bedside momentarily so that the nurse can speak with her. Support of the grieving family is important at this time. Identify three interventions the nurse may use to support Mrs. Oishi.

9. Indicate whether each of the following statements is true or false.

a. _____ At the time of a patient's death, federal law requires identification of potential organ or tissue donors.

b. _____ It is the nurse's responsibility to ask permission for an autopsy.

c. _____ During the care of the body after death, it is important to remove the patient's dentures.

d. _____ While the body is being prepared, name tags are placed on the body to identify it.

e. _____ At the time of death, the family must know who among them can legally give consent for organ donation.

Exercise 2

 CD-ROM Activity

 30 minutes

 In this exercise you will visit Harry George, a 54-year-old Caucasian male who was admitted to the hospital with symptoms of infection and swelling of the foot. He has a history of abusing alcohol. He has been diagnosed with cellulitis and osteomyelitis of the foot. You may have worked with Harry George previously if you already completed Lesson 1, 16, or 18.

• Sign in to work at Pacific View Regional Hospital on the Medical-Surgical Floor for Period of Care 1. (*Note:* If you are already in the virtual hospital from a previous exercise, click on **Leave the Floor** and then **Restart the Program** to get to the sign-in window.)
• From the Patient List, select Harry George (Room 401).
• Click on **Get Report**.
• Click on **Go to Nurses' Station**.
• Click on **Chart** and then on **401**.
• Click on and review the **Nursing Admission**.
• Now click on and review the **History and Physical**.

1. Harry George has experienced different types of loss. Each are affected by the level of stress he has experienced. Describe a source of stress Harry George is experiencing for each of the factors below.

Situational

Maturational

Sociocultural

2. A focused assessment will help the nurse better understand the nature of stress affecting Harry George. For each of the assessment categories below, write two questions you would ask the patient.

Perception of stressor

Adherence to healthy practices

3. Below, describe both the actual and perceived losses experienced by Harry George.

Actual

Perceived

4. When the nurse is assessing a patient's stage of grief, it is important to assess how a

patient _____ reacting rather than how the patient should be reacting.

5. A person who becomes overwhelmed by grief and often takes on self-destructive behavior

   is experiencing _____ grief.

6. According to Bowlby's phases of mourning, the phase of _____ arouses emotional outbursts and acute distress.

7. _____ is defined as the anticipation of a continued good.

8. For each of the following dimensions, describe a nursing intervention that would realistically promote hope for Harry George.

Cognitive dimension

Behavioral dimension

Contextual dimension

LESSON 18

Self-Concept

OO **Reading Assignment:** Growth and Development (Chapter 21)
Self-Concept and Sexuality (Chapter 22)

Patients: Harry George, Medical-Surgical Floor, Room 401
Dorothy Grant, Obstetrics Floor, Room 201

Objectives:

- Identify the components of self-concept.
- Describe stressors that affect self-concept of patients in the case studies.
- Discuss the influence of a nurse's behavior on a patient's self-concept.
- Apply the critical thinking model to assessment of a patient's self-concept.
- Develop a concept map for a case study patient with self-concept alterations.
- Describe the nursing diagnostic process for a patient with alteration in self-concept.
- Identify interventions useful in the promotion of self-concept.

Overview:

The self-concept is a complex mixture of thoughts, attitudes, and perceptions that shape how a person thinks about himself or herself. A person's self-concept affects all situations and relationships with others in addition to that person's own self-esteem. Disease, injury, and resultant disability all can threaten a person's self-concept and self-esteem. As a nurse, you play an important role in helping patients adapt to stressors caused by health alterations. What individuals think and how they feel about themselves affect the way they care for themselves physically and emotionally. Knowledge of variables that affect self-concept and approaches that promote self-concept will enable you to provide patients appropriate support and treatment.

Exercise 1

 CD-ROM Activity

 45 minutes

 In this exercise you will visit Harry George, a 54-year-old Caucasian male who was admitted to the hospital with symptoms of infection and swelling of the foot. He has a history of abusing alcohol. He has been diagnosed with cellulitis and osteomyelitis of the foot. You may have worked with Harry George previously if you already completed Lesson 1, 16, or 17.

- Sign in to work at Pacific View Regional Hospital on the Medical-Surgical Floor for Period of Care 3. (*Note:* If you are already in the virtual hospital from a previous exercise, click on **Leave the Floor** and then **Restart the Program** to get to the sign-in window.)
- From the Patient List, select Harry George (Room 401).
- Click on **Get Report**.
- Click on **Go to Nurses' Station**.
- Click on **Chart** and then on **401**.
- Click on and review the **Nursing Admission**.
- Click on and review the physician's **History and Physical**.

1. Self-concept is always changing and developing. From the list below, identify those factors that have affected Harry George's self-concept since his motorcycle accident 4 years ago. Select all that apply.

_____ Sense of competency

_____ Perceived reaction of others to his body

_____ Employment-related identity

_____ Perceptions of events that have affected self

_____ Racial identity

_____ Self-expectations

2. Explain how the loss of employment has likely affected Harry George's self-concept.

 3. Of the following developmental stages of life described by Erik Erikson, which is most likely disrupted in the case of Harry George? (*Study Tip:* Review Erikson's theory on page 584 in your textbook.)
   a. Integrity versus despair
   b. Industry versus inferiority
   c. Initiative versus guilt
   d. Generativity versus self-absorption and stagnation

➜ • Now click on **Consultations**.
   • Review the Psychiatric Consult.
   • Review the Mental Health Summary.

4. A self-concept stressor threatens a person's identity, body image, and role performance. Match each of Harry George's stressors below with the appropriate self-concept category.

Harry George's Stressors	Self-Concept Categories
_____ Impotence	a. Body image
_____ Loss of role as husband	b. Identity
_____ Emotional depression	c. Role performance
_____ Failure to maintain personal grooming	
_____ Job loss	
_____ Chronic wound	
_____ Seen as a public nuisance	

5. The expectations of family and friends on how Harry George should have behaved immediately following his injury would be described as a _____ role.

6. Harry George's _____ image involves attitudes he has about his appearance, impotence, and the effects of his diabetes.

7. Harry George's emotional appraisal of himself as a "loser" is a form of self-evaluation described as _____ esteem.

8. Harry George's _____ performance is the way in which he perceives his ability to be competent as a parent.

9. Developing a nursing diagnosis when a patient has an alteration in self-concept is complex. Often an assessment finding can be a defining characteristic for more than one nursing diagnosis. The defining characteristics from Harry George's data are listed below. Complete the concept map by writing the letter of each defining characteristic under the appropriate nursing diagnosis(es). (*Note:* A defining characteristic may be used for more than one diagnosis.)

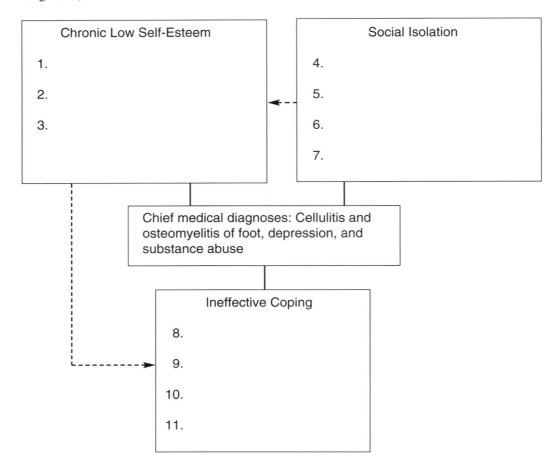

Defining Characteristics:

a. Sleep disturbance
b. Expression of shame/guilt
c. Change in communication pattern/uncommunicative
d. Abuse of chemical agent
e. Exists in a subculture
f. Inability to meet basic needs
g. Sad affect
h. Poor or no eye contact
i. Self-negating verbalization

10. Harry George is a complex case. Given the nursing diagnoses of Chronic Low Self-Esteem, Social Isolation, and Ineffective Coping, which would likely be your priority? Explain.

Exercise 2

 CD-ROM Activity

 45 minutes

 In this exercise you will visit Dorothy Grant, a pregnant 25-year-old Caucasian patient who was admitted to the hospital after blunt trauma to the abdomen. You may have worked with Dorothy Grant previously if you already completed Lesson 4.

- Sign in to work at Pacific View Regional Hospital on the Obstetrics Floor for Period of Care 1. (*Note:* If you are already in the virtual hospital from a previous exercise, click on **Leave the Floor** and then **Restart the Program** to get to the sign-in window.)
- From the Patient List, select Dorothy Grant (Room 201).
- Click on **Get Report**.
- Click on **Go to Nurses' Station**.
- Click on **Chart** and then on **201**.
- Click on and review the **History and Physical**.
- Click on and review the **Nursing Admission**.

1. As a victim of abuse, Dorothy Grant faces many factors that threaten her self-concept. Her concern for her unborn baby and her other children creates stress on her ability to function as a wife and mother. Application of critical thinking will ensure a more comprehensive assessment of this patient's situation. Complete the following critical thinking diagram for assessment of Dorothy Grant's situation by writing the letter of each critical thinking factor under its proper category.

Knowledge

1. _____

2. _____

3. _____

Experience   **ASSESSMENT SELF-CONCEPT**   **Attitudes**

4. _____

5. _____

6. _____

Standards

7. _____

8. _____

9. _____

Critical Thinking Factors

a. Consider your own feelings if, as a parent, you have ever believed your children were at risk.
b. Ask Dorothy Grant, "You said you want to be a good mother. Tell me what you mean by that."
c. Review concepts on domestic violence.
d. While caring for Dorothy Grant, apply what you have learned in caring for other victims of abuse.
e. While assessing Dorothy Grant, reinforce that any decisions about getting help to leave her husband will be her decisions only.
f. Consider concepts about self-esteem as you assess Dorothy Grant's needs.
g. Ask Dorothy Grant to tell her story by saying, "Tell me how your relationship with your husband has changed since you first married."
h. Ask the patient whether you can talk with her sister about her relationship with her children.
i. Apply principles of communication and caring while establishing a therapeutic relationship with Dorothy Grant.

• Click on **Return to Nurses' Station**.
- Click on **Leave the Floor**.
- Click on **Restart the Program**.
- Sign in to work at Pacific View Regional Hospital on the Obstetrics Floor for Period of Care 3.
- From the Patient List, select Dorothy Grant (Room 201).
- Click on **Get Report**.
- Click on **Go to Nurses' Station**.
- Click on **201** at bottom of screen.
- Click on **Patient Care** and then **Nurse-Client Interactions**.
- Select and view the video titled **1500: Managing Preterm Labor**. (*Note:* Check the virtual clock to see whether enough time has elapsed. You can use the fast-forward feature to advance the time by 2-minute intervals if the video is not yet available. Then click again on **Patient Care** and **Nurse-Client Interactions** to refresh the screen.)

2. List three nursing behaviors observed during the video interaction that reflect the nurse's acceptance of Dorothy Grant.

3. Identify three self-concept issues that a nurse should clarify about himself or herself when caring for patients.

 • Click on **Chart** and then on **201**.
- Select **Consultations**.
- Review the psychiatric and social work notes.

4. The information from Dorothy Grant's medical record provides considerable information about her health problems. Complete the diagnostic process chart below.

Assessment Activities	Defining Characteristics	Nursing Diagnosis
Observe patient's nonverbal behaviors	During admission seen crying and wringing hands	_____
Observe patient's self-report of situation	Reports being scared	
Ask about decisions made or test ability to problem-solve	Reports decisions are deferred to husband	
_____	States she is unable to please husband	Situational low self-esteem
_____	"I'm scared. What am I going to do?"	
Ask patient to describe how she feels about situation	" _____ _____ "	

5. For the diagnosis of Situational Low Self-Esteem, list three interventions you would plan for Dorothy Grant and give a rationale for each.

In questions 6 through 8, fill in the blanks describing aspects of evaluation of care.

6. In evaluating a plan of care, you apply knowledge of behaviors and characteristics of a healthy _____ when you review behaviors your patient displays.

7. Key indicators of a patient's self-concept can be _____ behaviors.

8. If your plan of care involved teaching Dorothy Grant about the risks and outcomes of domestic violence, you would evaluate her ability to _____ or _____ issues pertaining to domestic violence, indicating her level of _____.

LESSON 19

Principles Applied in Care of Older Adults

Reading Assignment: Health Assessment and Physical Examination (Chapter 15)
Administering Medications (Chapter 16)
Growth and Development (Chapter 21)
Safety (Chapter 27)

Patients: William Jefferson, Skilled Nursing Floor, Room 501
Clarence Hughes, Medical-Surgical Floor, Room 404
Pablo Rodriguez, Medical-Surgical Floor, Room 405

Objectives:

- Describe physiologic changes of aging.
- Identify common developmental tasks of older adults.
- Differentiate among dementia, delirium, and depression.
- Discuss older adult health concerns as they apply to patients in the case studies.
- Discuss safety risks as they apply to patients in the case studies.
- Apply critical thinking to the assessment of a patient's safety risks.
- Develop a plan of care for an older adult with safety risks.

Overview:

The care you provide older adults is challenging because of the normal variation in their physiologic, cognitive, and psychosocial health, as well as their functional ability. Most older adults are active and functionally independent despite the prevalence of chronic disease. However, there are those older adults who suffer from cognitive deficits and disease that result in various forms of disability. Because of the normal changes of aging being complicated by associated changes of chronic disease, the assessment of older adults can be difficult. As a nurse you must be able to understand the process of aging and not assume that all older adults have signs and symptoms representative of disease.

A major concern when caring for older adults is the ability to maintain a safe environment. Changes associated with aging increase patients' risk for falls and other accidents. As a nurse you are responsible for understanding a patients' risks for injury, anticipating their needs, and introducing preventive measures that ensure their safety and well-being.

Exercise 1

CD-ROM Activity

45 minutes

In this exercise you will visit William Jefferson, a 75-year-old African-American male who has a history of early Alzheimer's disease and who is now in the skilled nursing unit following admission to the hospital for a urinary tract infection and sepsis. You may have worked with William Jefferson previously if you already completed Lesson 11.

- Sign in to work at Pacific View Regional Hospital on the Skilled Nursing Floor for Period of Care 1. (*Note:* If you are already in the virtual hospital from a previous exercise, click on **Leave the Floor** and then **Restart the Program** to get to the sign-in window.)
- From the Patient List, select William Jefferson (Room 501).
- Click on **Get Report**.
- Click on **Go to Nurses' Station**.
- Click on **Chart** and then on **501**.
- Click on and review the **Nursing Admission**.

1. List four developmental tasks that pose difficulties for William Jefferson and give a rationale for each.

2. William Jefferson takes eight different medications ordered by his physician. Polypharmacy increases his risk for adverse drug reactions. Explain what you would do to ensure William Jefferson takes his medications safely and appropriately once he returns home. (*Study Tip:* Review pages 404 through 406 in your textbook.)

3. The nursing history reveals that William Jefferson has a hearing loss in the left ear. When considering hearing loss in older adults the nurse must recognize which of the following? (*Study Tip:* Review page 330 your textbook.)
a. Older adults are at an increased risk for hearing loss as a result of polypharmacy.
b. Older adults have difficulty distinguishing low-pitched sounds.
c. Thinning of the tympanic membrane is a source of hearing loss in the older adult.
d. Hearing consonants such as s, z, t, and g is increasingly difficult for older adults.

4. Indicate whether each of the following statements is true or false.

a. _____   Always speak toward the ear affected by the hearing loss.

b. _____   Check the ear canal for cerumen impaction.

c. _____   Speak in a clear, high-pitched tone at a higher volume.

d. _____   Reduce background noise during a discussion.

e. _____   Encourage patients to wear their hearing devices during a conversation.

➡ • Click on and review the **History and Physical**.

5. The record indicates that William Jefferson has experienced delirium.

a. What was the most likely cause of William Jefferson's delirium?

b. What other factors might have contributed to the delirium?

c. How does delirium differ from dementia in regard to onset, progression, orientation, and memory?

    d. Patients with Alzheimer's disease frequently also suffer depression. Depression can be distinguished from both dementia and delusions in what ways?

6. Nursing assessment of a patient with dementia and delirium is especially complex when the aging patient also suffers from chronic disease. Critical thinking applied to assessment enables a nurse to identify relevant nursing diagnoses. Complete the following critical thinking diagram for assessment of William Jefferson by writing the letter of each critical thinking factor under its proper category.

Knowledge

1. _____

2. _____

3. _____

Experience	**ASSESSMENT** **WILLIAM JEFFERSON**	**Standards**
4. _____		5. _____
		6. _____

Attitudes

7. _____

8. _____

Critical Thinking Factors

    a. Ask the patient's wife to describe how his sleep is affected when he becomes anxious or fearful.

    b. Consider the effects diabetes has on physical assessment findings for vascular and neurologic function.

    c. Reflect on previous encounters when you have assessed confused patients.

    d. Introduce yourself when you begin to assess William Jefferson and use a calm, steady approach, explaining each step with conviction.

    e. Refer to a gerontology text on the characteristics of dementia.

    f. Take time in assessing William Jefferson, do not rush, and examine all body systems thoroughly.

    g. Consider the effects William Jefferson's medications have on physical findings.

    h. When assessing his level of discomfort, always use a pain scale.

• Click on **Return to Nurses' Station**.
 • Select **501** at the bottom of the screen.
 • Review the **Initial Observation**.
 • Click on **Patient Care** and then on **Nurse-Client Interactions**.
 • Select and view the video titled **0730: Intervention—Patient Safety**. (*Note:* Check the virtual clock to see whether enough time has elapsed. You can use the fast-forward feature to advance the time by 2-minute intervals if the video is not yet available. Then click again on **Patient Care** and **Nurse-Client Interactions** to refresh the screen.)

7. William Jefferson presents several risk factors for falls. Complete the following fall assessment tool for this patient by identifying each of the clinical factors that apply to him. Select all that apply.

_____ History of falls

_____ Confusion

_____ Age (over 65)

_____ Impaired judgment

_____ Sensory deficit

_____ Unable to ambulate independently

_____ Decreased level of cooperation

_____ Increased anxiety

_____ Incontinence

_____ Medications affecting blood pressure or consciousness

_____ Postural hypotension with dizziness

8. Based on what you know about William Jefferson's condition, complete the following care plan for the nursing diagnosis Risk for Falls. Provide one goal, two expected outcomes, and three interventions relevant to this patient's situation.

Plan of Care Component

Goal

Expected Outcomes

1.

2.

Interventions

1.

2.

3.

9. Which of the following devices would be useful in protecting William Jefferson from falling as he gets out of bed?
    a. Vail enclosed bed
    b. Jacket restraint
    c. Ambularm
    d. Full set of side rails

An optimal goal for all patients is a restraint-free environment. For questions 10 through 14, fill in the blanks in the statements describing principles to follow when using restraints.

10. A _____ order is required for the application of a restraint.

11. If a nurse restrains a patient because of aggressive behavior, a face-to-face physician assessment is needed within _____ hour.

12. Always secure a restraint with a _____ tie.

13. Once applied, a restraint should be removed at least every _____ hours.

14. Restraints may be one of two categories. These categories are _____ and

    _____.

15. Which of the following may be complications associated with restraint use? Select all that apply.

    _____ Pressure ulcers

    _____ Strangulation

    _____ Pneumonia

    _____ Constipation

Exercise 2

 CD-ROM Activity

 30 minutes

 In this exercise you will visit Clarence Hughes, a 73-year-old African-American male with a several-year history of degenerative joint disease, osteoarthritis, and glaucoma. You may have worked with Clarence Hughes previously if you already completed Lesson 3.

- Sign in to work at Pacific View Regional Hospital on the Medical-Surgical Floor for Period of Care 1. (*Note:* If you are already in the virtual hospital from a previous exercise, click on **Leave the Floor** and then **Restart the Program** to get to the sign-in window.)
- From the Patient List, select Clarence Hughes (Room 404).
- Click on **Get Report**.
- Click on **Go to Nurses' Station**.
- Click on **Chart** and then on **404**.
- Click on and review the **History and Physical**.

1. Clarence Hughes reportedly has constipation.

   a. What normal physiologic change of aging might contribute to this problem?

   b. How might Clarence Hughes' osteoarthritis further contribute to constipation?

   c. What influences can medications associated with surgery and the postoperative phase have on Clarence Hughes' constipation?

2. Clarence Hughes has a history of smoking, which adds to the risks for respiratory problems. Below, identify the normal physical changes that occur in the respiratory system with aging. Select all that apply.

   _____ Increased number of alveoli

   _____ Decreased cough reflex

   _____ Decreased vital capacity

   _____ Increased removal of mucus

   _____ Increased airway resistance

   _____ Increased risk for respiratory infections

➡ • Now review the **Nursing Admission**.

3. Chronic disease diminishes the well-being of older adults. Identify three nursing interventions focusing on prevention that would be appropriate for Clarence Hughes based on his nursing admission data.

4. In order to encourage smoking cessation for Clarence Hughes, what type of intervention might you have to offer for him to be willing to stop smoking?

5. After reviewing Clarence Hughes' admission data, describe how he has been able to meet each of the following developmental tasks.

Maintaining quality of life

Redefining relationships with adult children

Exercise 3

 CD-ROM Activity

 30 minutes

 In this exercise you will visit Pablo Rodriguez, a 71-year-old Hispanic male who is suffering from advanced-stage lung cancer. You may have worked with Pablo Rodriguez previously if you already completed Lesson 6, 11, 12, or 13.

- Sign in to work at Pacific View Regional Hospital on the Medical-Surgical Floor for Period of Care 2. (*Note:* If you are already in the virtual hospital from a previous exercise, click on **Leave the Floor** and then **Restart the Program** to get to the sign-in window.)
- From the Patient List, select Pablo Rodriguez (Room 405).
- Click on **Get Report**.
- Click on **Go to Nurses' Station**.
- Click on **Chart** and then on **405**.
- Click on and review the **Nursing Admission**.

1. Pablo Rodriguez admits to being "mildly depressed." Indicate whether each of the following statements describing the features of depression is true or false.

   a. _____   Depression is typically worse in the evening hours.

   b. _____   Depression increases the safety risks for the older adult.

   c. _____   A person with depression usually has reduced awareness of activities around him.

   d. _____   The sleep-wake cycle is usually disturbed with depression, resulting in early morning awakening.

   e. _____   A person who is depressed is selectively disoriented.

➤ • Click on **Return to Nurses' Station**.
  • Click on **405** at the bottom of the screen to enter the patient's room.
  • Review the **Initial Observations**.
  • Click on **Patient Care** and then **Physical Assessment**.
  • Click on and review the assessment findings for the following categories: **Head & Neck**, **Chest**, **Upper Extremities**, and **Lower Extremities**.

2. Considering Pablo Rodriguez's physical findings, which of the following findings might be associated with a physiologic change of aging? Select all that apply.

   _____ Swollen gums

   _____ Cerumen in ear canal

   _____ Dry mouth

   _____ Impaired chest expansion

   _____ No adventitious sounds

   _____ Warm skin

   _____ Fair skin turgor

   _____ Muscle weakness

   _____ Swelling of leg

   _____ Skin dry

3. What factor in Pablo Rodriguez's history would complicate the physical findings you identified above?